10.25

Brigham and Women's Hospital Handbook of Diagnostic Imaging

Edited by

Barbara J. McNeil, M.D., Ph.D.
Professor of Radiology and Clinical Epidemiology,
Harvard Medical School; Radiologist and Director
of Center for Cost-Effective Care,
Brigham and Women's Hospital,
Boston, Massachusetts

Herbert L. Abrams, M.D.
Philip H. Cook Professor of Radiology,
Harvard Medical School; formerly, Chairman of Radiology,
Harvard Medical School and Brigham and Women's Hospital,
Boston, Massachusetts; Visiting Professor of Radiology,
Stanford University, Stanford,
California

**The Department of Radiology, Harvard Medical School,
and Brigham and Women's Hospital**

Foreword by Robert G. Petersdorf, M.D.
Vice Chancellor and Dean, University of California,
San Diego, School of Medicine, La Jolla,
California

Little, Brown and Company
Boston/Toronto

Library of Congress Catalog Card No. 85-81195

ISBN 0-316-56322-6

Printed in the United States of America

MV

This manuscript was prepared by health-care professionals who provide care to patients at the Brigham and Women's Hospital, Inc. in Boston, Massachusetts. This manuscript is not an official publication of the Brigham and Women's Hospital, Inc.

To the staff, residents, and fellows

of the Brigham and Women's Hospital

and Harvard Medical School

Contents

IV. Neurological Disease

V. Thyroid Disease

VI. Bone Disease

Appendixes

Foreword

This is an interesting little book for several reasons. First, it deals with a field of medicine that has literally exploded in logarithmic fashion. New imaging techniques are coming to the fore annually and often more frequently. What is the poor clinician to do when confronted with the maze of new information, most of which does not fall into his field of expertise? For diagnostic imaging, this little book provides most of the answers and when it does not, it tells us where to look.

Second, the book uses a sound problem-oriented approach. We are asked to think of clinical problems—masses, hypertension, trauma, hematuria, fractures—rather than in terms of technology. In other words, the book takes a strictly clinical point of view of imaging. Fortunately, it does not leave us with the picture of a technology looking for a job. Along similar lines, this book takes a broad view of diagnostic techniques. It is not afraid to compare imaging techniques with endoscopy and even physical examination.

Third, the book is brief and to the point. Its brevity, indeed its terseness, is a virtue found in few textbooks today. For those who want to know more there is an ample list of up-to-date references. For a broad-based general internist and infectious disease specialist like me, whose clinical terrain crosses all systems, there was just enough about new imaging techniques that I did not know, but was afraid to ask. For the occasional clinical theme on which I wanted to dwell in greater depth, there are one or two references to titillate my intellectual palate.

Fourth, the book is very much in the present. A nonradiologist in a non-system oriented specialty can use this book as a primer to play catch-up. I learned, for example, that scintiscans are superior to that old standby, the cholecystogram, in which I had been nurtured. For the first time I learned to put digital subtraction angiography into perspective *vis a vis* arteriography.

Fifth, the book is scrupulously honest. It does not attempt to glamorize diagnostic imaging. It tell us what techniques are most likely to be sensitive and which are most specific. It provides a fair picture of adverse reactions. Sometimes I wish there were a little more on cost-effectiveness, an arena in which the editors have made notable contributions. But the decision whether a hospital should invest in yet another CT scanner or in a digital subtraction angiography unit, or put itself in hock to magnetic imaging equipment, depends on factors such as the number of patients with a given problem, the case mix, and the availability of well-trained imaging personnel. These factors will differ widely from institution to institution. Besides, cost-effectiveness changes with time. I remember the early papers on CT scanning, which proposed that these machines be installed sparingly. Yet today there are few hospitals that do secondary and tertiary care that can afford to be without them. I guess we cannot expect to extrapolate the subject matter from a book directed at clinicians who have to make clinical decisions to the issues of how technology should be utilized.

Finally, this little book serves as a tribute to the Brigham and Women's Hospital, an institution which I once served as Chief Executive Officer. Along with other American teaching hospitals, the BWH is clearly a top-notch research hospital. It has pioneered much in investigation, both basic and applied. But as important as the Brigham's investigative advances are, it is its steadfast insistence on clinical excellence that makes it great. People who work there love to practice clinical medicine, not only well but also at the cutting edge. Only an institution such as the BWH, at which clinical medicine is held in high esteem, is capable of producing a book as full of clinical pearls as are contained in this small volume. This book is a credit, then, not only to its authors and editors, but also to the institution that spawned it.

I hope that other readers will have as much fun reading this book and learn as much from it as I did.

Robert G. Petersdorf, M.D.

Preface

Modern diagnostic imaging has undergone a revolution within the past three decades. Conventional radiologic procedures have been supplemented by a host of new methods, never before available. In the fifties and sixties, the development of angiography expanded our knowledge of the heart and the vascular bed of man. Lymphangiography in the early sixties permitted an assessment of lymphatic channels, of lymph node involvement, and of the mysteries of the retroperitoneum. Nuclear medicine in the seventies provided increasingly accurate information that combined images with functional data. Simultaneously, diagnostic ultrasound experienced a series of technologic breakthroughs that have led to a superior imaging method. Computed tomography in the seventies and eighties, and now nuclear magnetic resonance (NMR) imaging have transformed our approach to the diagnosis of disease in man by affording cross-sectional and/or digital imaging data of incomparably high quality.

Most physicians in practice today went through medical school long before many of the newer imaging techniques were applied. Some have been able to maintain a general familiarity with the changes that have occurred by a careful reading of the medical literature. But others have found themselves confused as to the proper use and sequence of imaging tests in a host of diseases with varying symptoms and signs. Furthermore, medical students entering the clinical arena confront a bewildering array of alternative methods, the capacities and limitations of which they are rarely fully aware.

As the methods have developed, there has been increasing concern about overutilization. This is particularly true of invasive procedures that have an irreducible number of complications. How do we weigh the impact of a procedure and the quality of the information it can reveal against its biological and monetary cost?

The conclusions outlined in this handbook represent the outgrowth of many years of grappling with such issues. Our desire was to produce a volume that would selectively and succinctly address the sequencing of current radiologic techniques in a reasonable number of important clinical settings.

We have not attempted to cover every sign or symptom confronted by the physician in practice. We have deliberately limited our approach to problems in which the new imaging modalities figure prominently, and in which clarification of their role in diagnosis or staging has seemed essential. The Brigham experience did not extend to the pediatric age group, an area that has been deliberately excluded.

To a major degree, this handbook is a product of living with medical problems on a day-to-day basis. A central part of each morning at the Brigham and Women's Hospital is the Medical/ X-ray Conference, at which the imaging studies of all in-patients are reviewed by a Senior Radiologist with the house staff and Senior Staff in Medicine responsible for the patients. Although the focus is on consultation and patient care, the conference has inevitably emerged as a central teaching vehicle as well. Time and again, examinations which simply were not indicated moved through the filtering process in Radiology to the point where their inappropriateness—and the mistaken basis for the initial request—could be fully and unequivocally discussed with the medical group.

This is, of course, a continuing education process. As each new group of house staff moves through the teaching hospital, they must be exposed to the appropriate use of complex diagnostic methods. The problem is more than that of efficient patient care. In the modern era, the whole system of prospective reimbursement is forcing referring physicians into patterns of choice that preclude the simultaneous ordering of a radionuclide examination, ultrasound, CAT scan, NMR, and angiography in the search for liver metastases. Both the health care system and the hospital would quickly move into bankruptcy were that to be done.

Rational choice is an essential part of the training of every physician—whether still in the learning stage, just beginning practice, or long in practice but unfamiliar with some of the new examinations now in use. This volume is a response, therefore, to those who have been concerned that they might be choosing examinations inappropriately, or following the wrong sequence, or subjecting their patients to unnecessary expense and radiation. In it we have distilled the experience of a large and expert pool of physicians both within and outside the Brigham and Women's Hospital.

Radiologists in the various specialized divisions of our department have provided the material for each of the sections in the *BWH Handbook,* and are clearly identified in those sections. In addition, Dr. Ferenc A. Jolesz has provided important information on magnetic resonance imaging. The algorithms and the accompanying text have also been reviewed by individuals outside of Radiology, and their responses and reactions have been invaluable. Each section has undergone a minimum of five revisions, the editors interacting with those who formulated the algorithms and the text initially, and with those who have critically reviewed the material. The end product represents an authoritative statement of the best sense of the Harvard/Brigham Department of Radiology faculty as to how examinations can be used most fruitfully, most economically, and most efficiently in clarifying the link between the underlying disease and the particular patient's signs and symptoms.

This book was written at a unique point in time, when magnetic resonance imaging had been introduced in clinical practice and yet was relatively unavailable at hospitals in this country. Not only was it inaccessible to most patients, but also the relative increment of diagnostic information afforded was not yet clearly defined. We have, therefore, chosen to base the algorithms on other, more widely available examinations and to indicate at the end of each section in a brief comment the likely contribution of NMR imaging as best we know it today. Within the next few years, prospectively designed assessments of the new technology will define its place in the chest and abdomen with far greater precision. At that point, the algorithms in this volume will be revised to take into account the changing face of medical diagnostic imaging.

The format of the *Handbook* reflects our desire to write a usable, pocket-sized volume that would be frequently consulted. Hence, we chose to make each chapter a combination of algorithm, text concerning the clinical situation and diagnostic examinations, and adequate references for supplementary information. We drew upon research and clinical insights. We acknowledge controversy and ambiguity, especially where a lack of adequate data affects numeric statements of sensitivity and specificity. In the appendix, we present current charges as listed by eight major medical institutions across the country for selective techniques referred to in the text, along with a list of radiation doses to critical organs, compiled by our BWH staff.

B.J.M.
H.L.A.

Introduction

The Algorithms

The key to each section is the algorithm, a kind of diagnostic decision tree, that indicates the most appropriate work-up for the patient with a given set of presenting symptoms and signs. In our journey through the algorithms, we often reach a "stop" sign, a point at which the diagnostic work-up is complete. Similarly, the final step is frequently "Rx," reflecting the satisfactory clarification of the problem so that proper management can and should be initiated.

Is ours the only way to go, the only correct sequence? Would that it were true! Manifestly, as in all of medicine, there are differences in background and experience that lead unalterably to special emphases. Aside from disparate perceptions as to the contribution of particular methods, the inherent ambiguity of medicine demands a variety of approaches. Nevertheless, it cannot be stated too often that our patterns of work-up represent a consensus rather than an individual approach. The consensus is simply not all-encompassing.

The Text

For each examination listed on the algorithm, its general qualities, drawbacks, sensitivity, and specificity are stated. We have walked a narrow tightrope between accessibility and ease of use of this handbook on the one hand, and comprehensiveness on the other. A great deal of pertinent information has been eliminated in the interests of making this a usable volume. If it were not immediately available to physicians concerned with a particular problem, it would represent a massive waste of time. Hence, the rather terse format and the somewhat dogmatic statements in some sections. Nevertheless, each section includes a list of articles to which the reader may refer for additional information.

In focusing on simplicity and clarity of presentation, we have not disregarded the uncertainty inherent at some of the branch points. An adequate data base has not always been available to document numeric statements of sensitivity and specificity. In such circumstances, the experience of our faculty and of others is reflected in such terms as "high," "moderately high," and "low," without actually indicating a percentage.

There is necessary repetition in the book. Under many of the algorithms, the same examination is included and described, so that the referring physician may look to the single symptom or sign with which he is concerned, without elaborate cross-referencing to other sections of the book. On rare occasions, the reader is referred to another section for a description of a method that has been used to clarify a similar problem.

The text begins with a description of a *typical patient,* by which we mean an individual whose symptoms and signs place him well within the category under discussion. This is followed by a telegraphic listing of the *typical disorders,* those which underlie the symptoms and signs with which the patient presents. Additional information concerning radiologic procedures or the clinical situation as a whole is included in a section on "Comments" at the beginning of the text.

The Examinations

In the order listed in the algorithms, each examination is described with a few pertinent comments as to its use, drawbacks, sensitivity, and specificity.

COMMENTS

These are features of the examination *as they relate to the clinical situation at hand.* They focus on the procedure's applicability and where possible compare it with other examinations.

DRAWBACKS

The information presented refers to the procedure's use in the specific setting. Complications, if any, are indicated in this section.

SENSITIVITY AND SPECIFICITY

As far as possible, these data are presented with reference to the specific clinical problem. When such information was not available, we have included the data we believed most relevant.

The traditional definitions of sensitivity and specificity as defined by the 2×2 decision matrix have been employed.

	Disease Present	Disease Absent
Test abnormal	a	c
Test normal	b	d
Total	a + b	c + d

Sensitivity (true positive ratio) = $a/(a+b)$
False negative ratio = $b/(a+b)$

Specificity (true negative ratio) = $d/(c+d)$
False positive ratio = $c/(c+d)$

Sensitivity is, therefore, the proportion of diseased individuals with abnormal tests; and specificity is the proportion of normal individuals with normal tests. When possible, we have tried to complement data on sensitivity and specificity with the best explanations for false positive and false negative examinations. Our list is not inclusive but is intended to help the reader apply the results in a more specific manner to a particular patient. In a few instances, we have also been able to provide information on a test's ability to provide information on differential diagnosis (e.g., benign versus malignant, cyst versus solid). Hopefully, future research will allow us to amplify this section of the text.

Ideally, we would have presented not just sensitivity and specificity data but probability data that would have allowed the clinician to know the *chance* that the patient had the disease in question *given* the occurrence of a positive or negative test. Such information requires knowledge of the prior clinical estimate of disease. This is generally patient specific and seemed too difficult to provide in a format sufficiently general to match the varied types of readers. In a few sections in which it seemed reasonable, we have presented such information.

Using the *Handbook*

The *BWH Handbook of Diagnostic Imaging* was designed for pocket use. Confronted with a patient who shows the symptoms and/or signs of spinal disease, the physician begins with a clinical suspicion as to their etiology. As the history, physical examination, and laboratory data come together to suggest more clearly a potential diagnosis, the need for diagnostic imaging data to rule out or verify that diagnosis is the trigger that sends the referring physician to the manual.

At that point, he must review the algorithm and determine at which point his patient enters. He may note that a bone scan has been requested, and both the rationale for that exam and its potential yield in the clinical situation will be readily available to him as he turns to the examination section and reviews the features, drawbacks, sensitivity, and specificity. If the bone scan is clearly positive, it may signal the end of the diagnostic imaging work-up. The diagnosis has been clarified, and the patient may now be treated appropriately. If the bone scan is negative or indeterminate—in chronic spinal cord compression, for example—the flow chart will carry him to the next step, namely computed tomography of the spine. Turning to the description of this test, he will understand readily why it is applicable at that point. He will also have a solid grasp of the degree to which a negative examination in the face of a high clinical suspicion may represent a false negative, and he is then able to adjust his confidence level to the established yield of the examination.

With time, and increased use of the manual, the referring physician will find it progressively more valuable. Finally, in any situation where more information is required than could be compressed into this terse monograph, the available references provide the reader with detailed analyses both of the examinations and the manner in which they have been applied to large groups of patients.

Acknowledgments

In a collective enterprise such as this, it is impossible to recognize fully the contributions that all have made. In a real sense, the book is dedicated to the residents and staff of the Harvard/Brigham Department of Radiology who have stimulated us to bring this information together. At still another level, the residents and staff of all of the other departments in the hospital have played a provocative and constantly prodding role in hundreds of thousands of clinical interactions over the years.

Those directly responsible for each of the sections are clearly indicated in the table of contents. Beyond that group, however, many individuals have participated in the review and analysis of much of the material in this book.

The following friends and colleagues have been immensely helpful: S. James Adelstein, Malcolm Bagshaw, Turner E. Bynum, Ronald A. Castellino, Victor M. Haughton, Bruce Hillman, Roland H. Ingram, James H. Maguire, Henry J. Mankin, Henry D. Royal, John Shillito, and Glenn D. Steele. Others who provided valuable information were: Daniel Bernstein, William D. Bloomer, Nathan P. Couch, Kenneth R. Falchuk, Harry Genant, P. Reed Larsen, Stephen J. Lipson, W. Bradford Patterson, David S. Rosenthal, Norman L. Sadowsky, Richard Scott, Barry A. Siegel, Thomas S. Thornhill, C. C. Wang, and Gordon H. Williams.

Without the intelligence, the drive, organization and commitment of Barbara Feinberg, this volume would never have been completed. She has played a critical role not alone in the organization of much of the material, but as an interface between editors and the section authors at each step in the process. Robbie Lauter has spent many hours of efficient work in bringing rough sections to an appropriate level of readability. Jo-Anne Polak was important in gathering the data on costs and Howard Stone and Susan Ross in gathering some of the older literature. Philip Judy and Robert Zimmerman have been responsible for the entire section on radiation dose. Jeffery Stoia has brought her sharp eye and superb critical judgment to a review of the galleys and page proofs that provided solid reassurance to the editors on the completion of their own concurrent review. Katherine Arnoldi supervised and coordinated the editorial process for Little, Brown in a manner that facilitated and assured the production of a fine volume. Curtis Vouwie, Senior Editor of the Medical Book Division of Little, Brown and Company, and many others at Little, Brown have provided support, encouragement, and quality editing that have contributed immeasurably to the final product.

To all, we extend our warm appreciation.

Contributing Authors

Douglass F. Adams, M.D.
Professor of Radiology, Harvard Medical School; Director, Division of Magnetic Resonance Imaging, Brigham and Women's Hospital, Boston, Massachusetts

Piran Aliabadi, M.D.
Visiting Associate Professor of Radiology, Harvard Medical School; Visiting Radiologist, Brigham and Women's Hospital, Boston, Massachusetts

Ross S. Berkowitz, M.D.
Associate Professor of Obstetrics and Gynecology, Harvard Medical School; Associate Director of Gynecologic Oncology, Brigham and Women's Hospital, Boston, Massachusetts

Michael A. Bettmann, M.D.
Associate Professor of Radiology, Harvard Medical School; Radiologist, Brigham and Women's Hospital, Boston, Massachusetts

Lawrence M. Boxt, M.D.
Assistant Professor of Radiology, Harvard Medical School; Radiologist, Brigham and Women's Hospital, Boston, Massachusetts

John M. Braver, M.D.
Assistant Professor of Radiology, Harvard Medical School; Co-Director, Division of Abdominal Imaging and Radiologist, Brigham and Women's Hospital, Boston, Massachusetts

T. Edward Bynum, M.D.
Associate Professor of Medicine, Harvard Medical School; Director of Clinical Gastroenterology, Brigham and Women's Hospital, Boston, Massachusetts

Peter M. Doubilet, M.D., Ph.D.
Assistant Professor of Radiology and Clinical Epidemiology, Harvard Medical School; Radiologist and Acting Director of Ultrasound Division, Brigham and Women's Hospital, Boston, Massachusetts

David E. Drum, M.D.
Associate Professor of Radiology, Harvard Medical School; Physician and Radiologist (Nuclear Medicine), Brigham and Women's Hospital, Boston, Massachusetts

George F. Edeburn, M.D.
Clinical Fellow in Radiology, Harvard Medical School; Resident in Radiology (Nuclear Medicine), Brigham and Women's Hospital, Boston, Massachusetts

Thomas J. Ervin, M.D.
Formerly, Assistant Professor of Medicine, Harvard Medical School, Boston, Massachusetts; Attending Physician in Hematology-Oncology, Maine Medical Center, Portland, Maine

Robert P. Fortunato, M.D.
Formerly, Instructor in Radiology, Harvard Medical School and Associate Radiologist, Brigham and Women's Hospital, Boston, Massachusetts

H. Harris Funkenstein, M.D.
Assistant Professor of Neurology, Harvard Medical School; Physician (Medicine), Brigham and Women's Hospital, Boston, Massachusetts

Stuart C. Geller, M.D.
Instructor in Radiology, Harvard Medical School; Assistant Radiologist, Massachusetts General Hospital, Boston, Massachusetts

Robert A. Greenes, M.D., Ph.D.
Associate Professor of Radiology, Harvard Medical School; Radiologist, Brigham and Women's Hospital, Boston, Massachusetts

Hani A. F. Haykal, M.D.
Instructor in Radiology, Harvard Medical School; Associate Radiologist, Brigham and Women's Hospital, Boston, Massachusetts

Maxine S. Jochelson, M.D.
Assistant Professor of Radiology, Harvard Medical School; Director, Division of Oncoradiology, Dana-Farber Cancer Institute; Radiologist, Brigham and Women's Hospital, Boston, Massachusetts

Ferenc A. Jolesz, M.D.
Assistant Professor of Radiology, Harvard Medical School; Radiologist, Brigham and Women's Hospital, Boston, Massachusetts

Philip F. Judy, Ph.D.
Assistant Professor of Radiology, Harvard Medical School; Associate in Radiology (Physics), Brigham and Women's Hospital, Boston, Massachusetts

William D. Kaplan, M.D.
Associate Professor of Radiology, Harvard Medical School; Chief, Oncologic Nuclear Medicine, Dana-Farber Cancer Institute; Radiologist (Nuclear Medicine), Brigham and Women's Hospital, Boston, Massachusetts

David C. Levin, M.D.
Professor of Radiology, Harvard Medical School; Acting Chairman of Radiology, Co-Director of Cardiovascular Radiology, Brigham and Women's Hospital, Boston, Massachusetts

Michael L. Lewis, M.D., Ph.D.
Formerly, Instructor in Radiology, Harvard Medical School; Director,

Magnetic Resonance Imaging and Neuroradiology, Houston Imaging Center, Houston, Texas

Robert J. Mayer, M.D.
Associate Professor of Medicine, Harvard Medical School; Associate Physician, Dana-Farber Cancer Institute, Boston, Massachusetts

Barbara J. McNeil, M.D., Ph.D.
Professor of Radiology and Clinical Epidemiology, Harvard Medical School; Radiologist and Director of Center for Cost-Effective Care, Brigham and Women's Hospital, Boston, Massachusetts

Harry Z. Mellins, M.D.
Professor of Radiology, Harvard Medical School; Director of Diagnostic Radiology, Brigham and Women's Hospital, Boston, Massachusetts

Michael F. Meyerovitz, M.B.B.Ch.
Instructor in Radiology, Harvard Medical School; Associate Radiologist, Brigham and Women's Hospital, Boston, Massachusetts

Daniel H. O'Leary, M.D.
Assistant Professor of Radiology, Harvard Medical School; Attending Radiologist, Brigham and Women's Hospital; Director of Carotid Noninvasive Laboratories, New England Deaconess Hospital, Boston, Massachusetts

Robert D. Pugatch, M.D.
Associate Professor of Radiology, Harvard Medical School; Director, Division of Thoracic Radiology, Brigham and Women's Hospital, Boston, Massachusetts

Jerome P. Richie, M.D.
Associate Professor of Urological Surgery, Harvard Medical School; Chief, Urologic Oncology, Brigham and Women's Hospital, Boston, Massachusetts

Calvin L. Rumbaugh, M.D.
Professor of Radiology, Harvard Medical School; Director, Division of Neuroradiology, Brigham and Women's Hospital, Boston, Massachusetts

Steven E. Seltzer, M.D.
Assistant Professor of Radiology, Harvard Medical School; Director, Division of Computed Tomography and Co-Director, Division of Abdominal Imaging, Brigham and Women's Hospital, Boston, Massachusetts

J. Leland Sosman, M.D.
Assistant Professor of Radiology, Harvard Medical School; Radiologist, Brigham and Women's Hospital, Boston, Massachusetts

Paul W. Spirn, M.D.
Instructor in Radiology, Harvard Medical School; Associate

Radiologist, Brigham and Women's Hospital, Boston, Massachusetts

Vera L. Stewart, M.D.
Instructor in Radiology, Harvard Medical School; Associate
Radiologist, Brigham and Women's Hospital, Boston, Massachusetts

Paul C. Stomper, M.D.
Instructor of Radiology, Harvard Medical School; Associate
Radiologist, Dana-Farber Cancer Institute and Brigham and
Women's Hospital, Boston, Massachusetts

Roger A. Styles, M.D.
Formerly, Clinical Fellow in Radiology, Harvard Medical School and
Clinical Fellow in Radiology (CT/US), Brigham and Women's
Hospital, Boston, Massachusetts; Radiologist, Wausau Medical
Center, Wausau, Wisconsin

Sabah S. Tumeh, M.D.
Assistant Professor of Radiology, Harvard Medical School; Associate
Radiologist, Brigham and Women's Hospital, Boston, Massachusetts

Dana A. Twible, M.D.
Formerly, Instructor in Radiology, Harvard Medical School and
Associate Radiologist, Brigham and Women's Hospital, Boston,
Massachusetts; Radiologist, Washington Hospital Center,
Washington, D.C.

Ay-Ming Wang, M.D.
Assistant Professor of Radiology, Harvard Medical School;
Radiologist, Brigham and Women's Hospital, Boston, Massachusetts

Barbara N. Weissman, M.D.
Associate Professor of Radiology, Harvard Medical School;
Radiologist and Director, Bone Radiology Service, Brigham and
Women's Hospital, Boston, Massachusetts

Amir A. Zamani, M.D.
Assistant Professor of Radiology, Harvard Medical School; Associate
Radiologist, Brigham and Women's Hospital, Boston, Massachusetts

Robert E. Zimmerman, M.S.E.E.
Principal Research Associate, Harvard Medical School; Associate in
Radiology (Physics), Brigham and Women's Hospital, Boston,
Massachusetts

Brigham and Women's Hospital
Handbook of Diagnostic Imaging

Abdominal Disease

Acute Abdominal Distress

Robert P. Fortunato

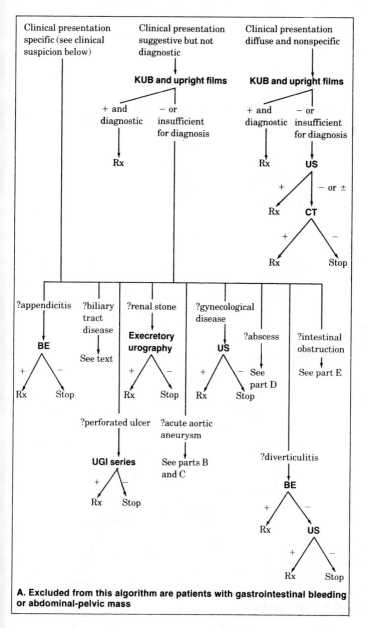

A. Excluded from this algorithm are patients with gastrointestinal bleeding or abdominal-pelvic mass

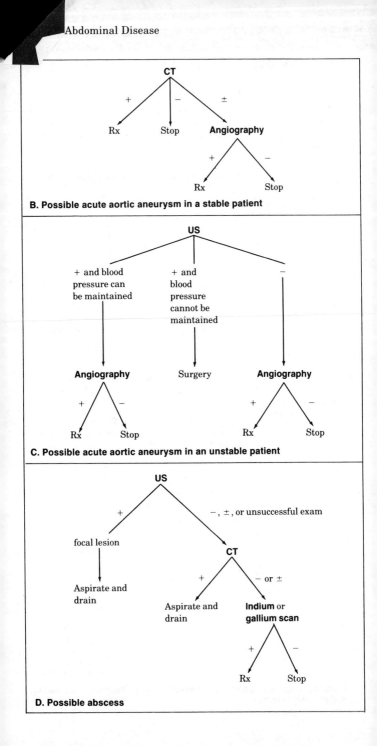

B. Possible acute aortic aneurysm in a stable patient

C. Possible acute aortic aneurysm in an unstable patient

D. Possible abscess

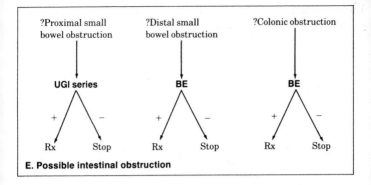

E. Possible intestinal obstruction

Typical Patient

Individual experiencing acute abdominal pain, discomfort, or distention, without gastrointestinal (GI) bleeding or discrete mass; includes postsurgical patients

Typical Disorder(s)

Diverticulitis
Appendicitis
Gastric/duodenal ulcer
Abscess
Acute aortic aneurysm
Renal stone
Intestinal obstruction (small bowel and colonic)

Plain Films (KUB and Upright)

Good screen for masses, distention of bowel loops, organomegaly
Demonstrates presence, location, and size of masses
Readily defines calcified masses
Orients further imaging examinations

Comments

Abnormal for about 10% of American patients with abdominal pain [4] and up to about 50% of British patients [15]; the worse the pain and tenderness, the greater the chance for positive radiographs [4]. Most frequent signs are for bowel obstruction, calculi, gallstones, or ileus [4].

Sensitivity

With local ileus or appendicolith as a sign of acute appendicitis: *40%* [15]
Having two abnormal findings in abdomen: *75%* [22]
With calculi as a sign of acute cholecystitis; *25%* [13]

With distended small bowel or gas-fluid levels as signs of small bowel obstruction: approaching *100%* [15]

Specificity

The signs on plain radiograph are relatively nonspecific and can apply to a number of diseases in acute or chronic (e.g., calculi) phases

Ultrasound (US)

Provides a broad range of imaging information
Useful screen when source of distress is uncertain
Defines presence, location, and size of masses
Distinguishes cystic from solid masses

Drawbacks

Intestinal gas can obscure visualization
Extra body fat impedes examination

Sensitivity

For abdominal abscess in patients with abdominal symptoms: about *80%* [7] and occasionally reported higher, *90%* [21]
   Sensitivity is generally less than that of CT
For pelvic abscesses: greater than *95%* [21]
False negatives can occur
   If surgical wounds prevent complete examination
   Less frequently in upper abdomen, where there are fewer obscuring bowel gas patterns [17]

Specificity

For suspected abscesses: about *90%* [7, 17] and occasionally reported higher, greater than *95%* [21]
   Specificity is generally less than that of CT

Computed Tomography (CT)

Provides a broad range of information
Precisely delineates mass and adjacent nodes, if present
Provides better resolution than ultrasound
Bowel gas does not interfere with the examination

Drawbacks

Rare complications; occasional contrast reactions and/or secondary renal failure occur, with serious reactions only 1 in 14,000 [2]

Comment

Examination is nonspecific and frequently noncontributory when intrinsic gastrointestinal disease is the source of abdominal distress

Sensitivity

For abdominal abscess in patients with abdominal symptoms: greater than *95%* [7, 12, 13, 17, 19, 24]
False negatives can occur
 If abscesses resemble bowel loops
For abdominal aortic aneurysms: approaching *100%* [1]
For defining caudal and cranial extent of aortic aneurysms in relation to renal arteries: approaching *100%* [1]

Specificity

For patients suspected of having abscesses: *85–95%* (the higher range more frequent) [7, 12, 13, 17, 19, 24]
False positives can occur
 If bowel loops simulate lesions (infrequently)
 In the presence of tumors with central necrosis, or thick-walled cysts
For patients suspected of having aortic aneurysms: no exact data, but probably about *90%*

Barium Enema (BE), Upper Gastrointestinal (UGI) Series

Primary approach to pathology involving the upper GI tract, small intestine, and colon
Frequently definitive
Positive results help orient medical or surgical management
Appendicitis is usually diagnosed clinically; in atypical clinical presentations, however, a barium enema may be helpful in a small percentage of cases

Drawbacks

In cases of bowel obstruction, long delays due to slow transit time of barium
Barium given orally with colonic obstruction can cause inspissation behind the obstruction (rare)

Sensitivity

UGI series
 For peptic disease and obstruction: high
Barium enema
 For appendicitis and diverticulitis without abscess: low
 For colonic obstruction and diverticulitis with abscess: high
False negatives can occur
 If diagnosis depends on passage of barium through the region of questioned obstruction, failure to obtain delayed films may preclude a correct diagnosis

Specificity

Barium enema: high
UGI series: high

False positives can occur
> Because spasm can occasionally simulate obstruction
> With inadequate follow-up for UGI series: filming must continue up to 24 hours post ingestion

Excretory Urography

Evaluates the upper urinary tract (kidneys and ureters) when associated injury to this area is suspected
May also allow examination of lower urinary tract if there is sufficient bladder distention

Drawbacks

Only about 15% of bladder injuries will be detected because of the failure to achieve adequate distention

Sensitivity

For renal injury: *87%*
For ureteral injuries (when combined with retrograde pyelography, if necessary): very high

Specificity

No precise data, but generally high

Angiography

Precisely defines vascular causes of acute abdominal distress and mass lesions, including aneurysm
Sole method of definitive diagnosis of acute ischemic bowel disease

Drawbacks

Complications: contrast reaction and/or secondary renal failure, rare; vascular injury and thrombosis, serious, about 1%; local hemorrhage or hematoma, nonfatal serious reactions, less than 2%; fatalities, .03% [9]

Comments

Not intended as primary examination, unless aneurysm suspected
If leaking aneurysm is suspected and if diagnosis of aneurysm is confirmed by ultrasound or CT, angiography is performed only if patient's blood pressure can be maintained

Sensitivity

For abdominal aortic aneurysms: about *70%* [1]
False negatives can occur
> If aneurysm is filled by laminated thrombus

Specificity

For defining normal abdominal aortas: about *95%*

Gallium Scan

Useful for a variety of abdominal processes including those in the vertebrae
Gallium can be injected directly in the form of gallium citrate (i.e., in vitro incubation with white cells not required)

Drawbacks

Usually requires 24 hours between injection and imaging. Further delayed views are sometimes necessary to distinguish normal GI excretion from pathological processes.
All subsequent numbers decrease significantly unless imaging is done on Anger camera instead of rectilinear scanner

Sensitivity

For abdominal abscesses: *85–90%* [8, 11, 13, 17]
    Sensitivity is lower than CT, higher than ultrasound
False negatives can occur
    In the presence of infections of very short duration or fungal infections

Specificity

Lower than CT, about *90%* [8, 13, 20]; variations from *65%* [17] to *95%* [11]
False positives can occur because of
    Colonic activity
    Accumulation in coexisting tumors
    Inflammatory bowel disease
    Activity associated with recent (less than 2 weeks) surgical intervention
    Acute hematomas rarely, usually when infected

Indium Leukocyte Scan

Potentially more specific than gallium since leukocytes accumulate at infection sites
Best for acute processes generally less than 1½ weeks in duration; chronic processes may have well-defined wall without inflammatory response [12]
Does not localize in gut as gallium does

Drawbacks

Requires in vitro incubation of patient's (or compatible individual's) white blood cells
Indium is not FDA approved and not generally available

Sensitivity

For abdominal abscesses: about *86%* [12]
False negatives can occur
> In states that alter normal distribution of leukocytes (e.g., antibiotic therapy, hyperalimentation, hemodialysis)
> In abscesses without leukocytes (e.g., fungi, TB)

Specificity

About *95%* [13]
False positives can occur
> If agent accumulates in spleen or in accessory spleen
> With acute gastrointestinal bleeding
> With ischemic bowel disease and in ulcerative colitis
> With acute hematomas [23]

Contribution of Magnetic Resonance Imaging [3, 10, 14]

May elucidate abdominal distress due to vascular disease
Readily defines abdominal and pelvic fluid collections, cysts, and abscesses
In aortic aneurysm, demonstrates location, size, and wall thickness, relationship to renal and iliac arteries, thrombus within aneurysm
In leaking aneurysms, visualizes retroperitoneal hematoma

References

1. Andersen, P. E., Jr., and Lorentzen, J. E. Comparison of computed tomography and aortography in abdominal aortic aneurysms. *J. Comput. Assist. Tomogr.* 7:670, 1983.
2. Broderick, T. W. Contrast material reactions. In G. W. Friedland, R. Filly, and M. L. Goris (Eds.). *Uroradiology.* New York: Churchill Livingstone, 1983.
3. Ehman, R. L., Kjos, B. O., Hricak, H., et al. Relative intensity of abdominal organs in MR images. *J. Comput. Assist. Tomogr.* 9:315, 1985.
4. Eisenberg, R. L., Heineken, P., Hedgcock, M. W., et al. Evaluation of plain abdominal radiographs in the diagnosis of abdominal pain. *Ann. Intern. Med.* 97:257, 1982.
5. Fisher, M. F., and Rudd, T. G. In-111 labeled leukocyte imaging: False-positive study due to acute gastrointestinal bleeding. *J. Nucl. Med.* 24:803, 1983.
6. Forstrum, L. A., Morin, R. L. McCullough, J. et al. Indium-111 labeled leukocyte imaging: A review of 1178 studies. *J. Nucl. Med.* 24:101, 1983.
7. Halber, M. D., Daffner, R. H., Morgan, C. L., et al. Intra-abdominal abscess: Current concepts in radiologic evaluation. *AJR* 133:9, 1979.
8. Henkin, R. E. Gallium-67 in the Diagnosis of Inflammatory Disease. In P. B. Hoffer, C. Bekerman, and R. E. Henkin (Eds.). *Gallium-67 Imaging.* New York: Wiley, 1978. Pp. 65–83, 90–92.

9. Hessel, S. J. Complications of Angiography and Other Catheter Procedures. In H. L. Abrams (ed.). *Abrams Angiography: Vascular and Interventional Radiology* (3rd ed.). Boston: Little, Brown, 1983. Pp. 1041–1055.

10. Higgins, C. B., Goldberg, H., Hricak, H., et al. Nuclear magnetic resonance imaging of vasculature of abdominal viscera: Normal and pathologic features. *AJR* 140:1217, 1983.

11. Kaplan, W. D. Imaging of Inflammatory Lesions. In P. B. Schneider and S. Treves (Eds.). *Nuclear Medicine in Clinical Practice.* North Holland: Elsevier, 1978. Pp. 299–310.

12. Knochel, J. Q., Koehler, P. R., Lee, T. G., et al. Diagnosis of abdominal abscesses with computed tomography, ultrasound and ^{111}In leukocyte scans. *Radiology* 137:425, 1980.

13. Korobkin, M., Callen, P. W., Filly, R. A., et al. Comparison of computed tomography, ultrasonography and gallium-67 scanning in the evaluation of suspected abdominal abscess. *Radiology* 129:89, 1978.

14. Kressel, H. Y., Axel, L., Thickman, D., et al. NMR imaging of the abdomen at 0.12 T. Initial clinical experience with a resistive magnet. *AJR* 141:1179, 1983.

15. Lee, P. W. R. The plain x-ray in the acute abdomen: A surgeon's evaluation. *Br. J. Surg.* 63:763, 1976.

16. McNeil, B. J., Sanders, R., Alderson, P. O., et al. A prospective study of computed tomography, ultrasound, and gallium imaging in patients with fever. *Radiology* 139:647, 1981.

17. Moir, C., and Robins, R. E. Role of ultrasonography, gallium scanning and computed tomography in the diagnosis of intra-abdominal abscess. *Am. J. Surg.* 143:582, 1982.

18. Peters, A. M., Saverymuttu, S. H., Reavy, H. J., et al. Imaging of inflammation with indium-111 tropolonate labeled leukocytes. *J. Nucl. Med.* 24:39, 1983.

19. Quinn, M. J., Sheedy, P. F., II, Stephens, D. H., et al. Computed tomography of the abdomen in evaluation of patients with fever of unknown origin. *Radiology* 136:407, 1980.

20. Sfakianakis, G. N., Al-Sheikh, W., Heal, A., et al. Comparisons of scintigraphy with In-111 leukocytes and Ga-67 in the diagnosis of occult sepsis. *J. Nucl. Med.* 23:618, 1982.

21. Taylor, K. J. W., Wasson, J. F. M., de Graaff, C., et al. Accuracy of grey-scale ultrasound diagnosis of abdominal and pelvic abscess in 220 patients. *Lancet* 1:83, 1978.

22. Thorpe, J. A. C. The plain abdominal radiograph in acute appendicitis. *Ann. R. Coll. Surg. Engl.* 61:45, 1979.

23. Wing, V. W., Van Sonnenberg, E., Kopper, S., et al. Indium-111 labeled leukocyte localization in hematomas: A pitfall in abscess detection. *Radiology* 152:173, 1984.

24. Wolverson, M. K., Jagannadharao, B., Sundaram, M., et al. CT as a primary diagnostic method in evaluating intra-abdominal abscess. *AJR* 133:1089, 1979.

2

Acute Cholecystitis

Robert P. Fortunato

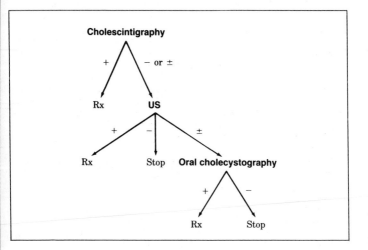

Typical Patient

Individual experiencing acute abdominal pain, right upper quadrant tenderness, fever, muscle spasm guarding, and occasionally slight jaundice

Typical Disorder(s)

Inflamed gallbladder, frequently (almost invariably) in association with calculi, or with a calculus occluding the cystic duct
Acute pancreatitis
Peptic ulcer disease
Hepatitis

Cholescintigraphy (^{99m}Tc-IDA Derivatives)

Highly sensitive and specific for acute state
Primary diagnostic approach
Available immediately, without need for contrast absorption through GI tract (as compared to oral cholecystogram)
Current agent (DISIDA—di-isopropyl iminodiacetic acid) can be used in patients with elevated bilirubin, up to 30 mg/dl

Comment

Requires a 3- to 6-hour fast

Sensitivity

Generally reported to be greater than *95%* [4, 8, 9]; occasionally lower [5]

False negatives can occur

> In the presence of acalculous cholecystitis, although in most patients (90%) there will be enough edema and inflammation occluding the cystic duct to prevent visualization of gallbladder

Specificity

Generally reported to be greater than *95%* [4, 8, 9], occasionally lower [6]

False positives can occur [3, 7]

> Without prior fasting or with prolonged fasting
> With alcoholism
> With total parenteral nutrition
> With acute pancreatitis
> With recent narcotics injection
> With hepatocellular disease

Ultrasound (US)

Provides good view of gallbladder wall

Gives useful information on right upper quadrant and on other viscera besides gallbladder

Helpful in differential diagnosis

Excellent at visualizing stones and estimating duct size

Drawbacks

Measures anatomy, not function; diagnosis of cholecystitis is only presumptive

Sensitivity

85–95% [1, 2, 4–6, 10]

False negatives can occur

> Without prior fasting
> With obesity
> If stone is mistaken for gas, polyp, or tumor

Specificity

Generally said to be greater than *90%* [1, 2, 4, 6], occasionally as low as *60%* [4]

Oral Cholecystography

Demonstrates gallbladder anatomy with high resolution

Drawbacks

Requires 12-hour delay, special diet, occasionally two doses over
    24 hours
Not good with elevated bilirubin, more than 2–4 mg/dl
Riskier for patients with myocardial infarction or renal failure
    because of renal toxicity of Telepaque

Comment

Rarely employed because of the quality of alternative examina-
    tions

Sensitivity

Highly variable: *30–90%* [4, 10]
False negatives can occur
    If stones are too small
    If stone is mistaken for gas, polyp, or tumor
    With suboptimal opacification
    If patient has diarrhea

Specificity

Not examination of choice, and few data are available
False positives can occur, however,
        For presence of stones
            If gas, polyp, tumor, or adenomyoma is mistaken for
                stone
        For presence of acute cholecystitis
            If patient fails to take medication
            If there is vomiting or diarrhea
            With gastric outlet obstruction
            With poor opacification

References

1. Bartrum, R. J., Jr., Crow, H. C., and Foote, S. R. Ultrasound examination of the gallbladder: An alternative to "double-dose" oral
   cholecystography. *JAMA* 236:1147, 1976.
2. Bartrum, R. J., Jr., Crow, H. C., and Foote, S. R. Ultrasonic and
   radiographic cholecystography. *N. Engl. J. Med.* 296:538, 1977.
3. Choy, D., Shi, E. C., McLean, R. G., et al. Cholescintigraphy in
   acute cholecystitis: Use of intravenous morphine. *Radiology*
   151:203, 1984.
4. Crade, M., Taylor, K. J. W., Rosenfield, A. T., et al. Surgical and
   pathologic correlation of cholecystosonography and cholecystography. *AJR* 131:227, 1978.
5. Freitas, J. E., Mirkes, S. H., Fink-Bennett, D. M., et al. Suspected
   acute cholecystitis. Comparison of hepatobiliary scintigraphy versus ultrasonography. *Clin. Nucl. Med.* 7:364, 1982.
6. Ralls, P. W., Colletti, P. M., Halls, J. M., et al. Prospective evaluation of ^{99m}Tc-IDA cholescintigraphy and gray-scale ultrasound in
   the diagnosis of acute cholecystitis. *Radiology* 144:369, 1982.

7. Serafini, A. N., Al-Sheikh, W., Barkin, J. S., et al. Biliary scintigraphy in acute pancreatitis. *Radiology* 144:591, 1982.
8. Weissmann, H. S., Badia, L., Sugarman, L. A., et al. Spectrum of 99m-Tc-IDA cholescintigraphic patterns in acute cholecystitis. *Radiology* 138:167, 1981.
9. Weissmann, H. S., Frank, M. S., Bernstein, L. H., et al. Rapid and accurate diagnosis of acute cholecystitis with ^{99m}Tc-HIDA cholescintigraphy. *AJR* 132:523, 1979.
10. Wolson, A. H., and Goldberg, B. B. Gray-scale ultrasonic cholecystography. A primary screening procedure. *JAMA* 240:2073, 1978.

3

Chronic Cholecystitis

Robert P. Fortunato

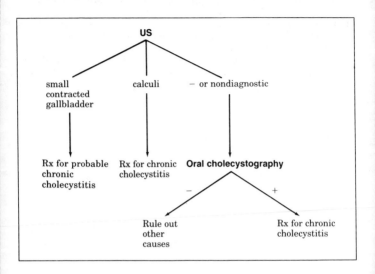

Typical Patient

Individual experiencing recurrent right upper quadrant pain

Typical Disorder(s)

Chronic cholecystitis
Peptic ulcer
Irritable bowel syndrome

Comments

In this algorithm there is no mention of cholescintigraphy,
which is more sensitive for determining the patency of the
cystic duct (and hence is better for the diagnosis of acute
cholecystitis) than for the presence of gallstones. In most patients with chronic cholecystitis, the gallbladder is visualized
(though frequently late) on cholescintigraphy. Quantitative
studies to measure gallbladder emptying (gallbladder "ejection fractions") have also been proposed, but data on their usefulness are limited and hence not discussed [5].

Some believe that gallstones per se do not imply clinically active
disease. If the reader believes this, then anatomical demonstration of gallstones (by ultrasound, for example) should not
lead to a diagnosis of chronic cholecystitis.

Ultrasound (US)

Visualizes the gallbladder
Gives ancillary data on right upper quadrant anatomy, including the normal hepatic duct (less than 4 mm) and obstructed hepatic duct (greater than 5 mm) [2]
Helpful in differential diagnosis
Rapid screen feasible

Drawbacks

Lower sensitivity and specificity in obese patients

Sensitivity

For detecting calculi: *96–98%* [1, 3, 4, 6]
False negatives can occur
> Without fasting
> With obese patients
> If stone is mistaken for gas, polyp, or tumor

Specificity

For showing normal gallbladder: *93–97%* [1, 3, 6]
False positives for gallstones can occur
> If stone is mistaken for gas, polyp, or tumor
False positives for chronic cholecystitis can occur
> If nonfasting state has led to small contracted gallbladder

Oral Cholecystography

Demonstrates calculi, but no better than ultrasound
Demonstrates gallbladder anatomy only if there is adequate concentration

Drawbacks

Covers a two-day period; 25% of patients need second dose of Telepaque [7]
Occasional renal reaction

Comment

Oral cholecystography has almost entirely been supplanted by ultrasound and computed tomography and is far less commonly performed than in the past

Sensitivity

92–94% [1]
False negatives for presence of stones can occur [8]
> If stones are too small or multiple
> With suboptimal opacification
> If patient has diarrhea or forgets to take Telepaque medication

Specificity

Few if any numerical data available; however, if the following false positive possibilities are ruled out, the specificity is high

False positives

    For presence of stones can occur

        If gas, polyp, tumor, or adenomyoma is mistaken for stone

    For presence of chronic cholecystitis can occur

        With liver failure

        If medication is not taken

        With vomiting/diarrhea

        With a gastric outlet obstruction

References

1. Berk, R. N., Ferrucci, J. T., Fordtran, J. S., Jr., et al. The radiological diagnosis of gallbladder disease. An imaging symposium. *Radiology* 141:49, 1981.
2. Cooperberg, P. L. High resolution real-time ultrasound in the evaluation of the normal and obstructed biliary tract. *Radiology* 129:477, 1978.
3. Cooperberg, P. L., Pon, M. S., Wong, P., et al. Real-time high resolution ultrasound in the detection of biliary calculi. *Radiology* 131:789, 1979.
4. Crade, M., Taylor, K. J. W., Rosenfield, A. T., et al. Surgical and pathologic correlation of cholecystosonography and cholecystography. *AJR* 131:227, 1978.
5. Krishnamurthy, G. T., Bobban, V. R., Kingston, E., et al. Measurement of gallbladder emptying sequentially using a single dose of 99mTc-labelled hepatobiliary agent. *Gastroenterology* 83:773, 1982.
6. McIntosh, D. M. F., and Penney, H. F. Gray-scale ultrasonography as a screening procedure in the detection of gallbladder disease. *Radiology* 136:725, 1980.
7. Mujahed, Z., Evans, J. A., and Whalen, J. P. The nonopacified gallbladder on oral cholecystography. *Radiology* 112: 1, 1974.
8. Palayew, M. J. Chronic cholecystitis and cholelithiasis. *Semin. Roentgenol.* 11:249, 1976.

Jaundice with Little or No Pain, Probable Obstruction, Possible Cancer

Douglass F. Adams

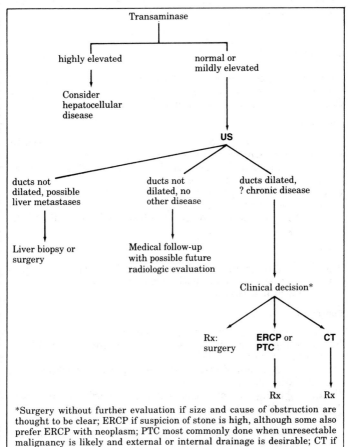

*Surgery without further evaluation if size and cause of obstruction are thought to be clear; ERCP if suspicion of stone is high, although some also prefer ERCP with neoplasm; PTC most commonly done when unresectable malignancy is likely and external or internal drainage is desirable; CT if suspicion of malignancy is high

Typical Patient

Individual with clinically apparent or chemical jaundice but experiencing minimal or no pain

Typical Disorder(s)

Pancreatic cancer

Primary hepatic disease (e.g., etiologies like hepatocellular dysfunction or intrahepatic cholestasis)

Cholangiocarcinoma

Comments

Older textbooks sometimes refer to patients with these symptoms as having "painless jaundice"

Ultrasound (US)

Defines presence or absence and degree of both intrahepatic and extrahepatic bile duct dilation

Better for visualizing head rather than tail or body of pancreas

Drawbacks

Pancreatic head or extrahepatic bile duct may be obscured by obesity or gastrointestinal air (38% of patients) [10]

Distinguishing acutely obstructed system from dilated nonobstructed system is difficult

Only about 23% of patients with acute obstruction caused by stones will show duct dilation [19]

Cause of obstruction is correctly determined only 23% of the time [9]

Comments

There is no particular area of obstruction (e.g., portal vs. suprapancreatic vs. infrapancreatic regions) in which ultrasound is superior at identifying site

Sensitivity

For detecting pancreatic disease: about *69%* [7]

For detecting pancreatic disease and identifying it as malignant or inflammatory: *56%* [7]

For detecting ducts dilated $\geq$ 6 mm in patients without prior biliary tract surgery: *90%* [17]

For determining level or site of obstruction (portal vs. suprapancreatic vs. infrapancreatic): wide variation, *30–60%* [9, 17]

False negatives for the site or etiology of obstruction can occur

  If obesity or gas prevents visualization of pancreas or common duct (5% of patients)

  If common duct stones are not visualized

  With dilated but nonobstructed ducts secondary to passed stone

Specificity

For diagnosing normal extrahepatic ducts (less than 6 mm) in patients without prior biliary tract surgery: *96%* [17]

For detecting normal pancreas: about *82%* [7]

False positives can occur if

  Surgical clips are mistaken for stone

Pancreatitis is mistaken for carcinoma
There has been prior biliary surgery [17]
Stone has recently been passed

Endoscopic Retrograde Cholangiopancreatography (ERCP)

Provides both diagnosis and location
Delineates pathology precise '
Success rate is 80–90% and i not dependent on dilated ducts [18]
Visualizes pancreatic duct
Sphincterotomy can be performed if necessary
Detects pancreatic cancer

Drawbacks

Cannulation and opacification of pancreatic duct occur in only 70% [13]
Cannulation and opacification of biliary system occur in only 46% [13]
Accurate less than half the time in detecting nonpancreatic lesions [13]

Sensitivity

For pancreatic tumor excluding failed cannulations: greater than *80%* [3, 5, 13]
For diagnosing site and cause of biliary obstruction: *85%* [9]
For diagnosing specific cause of jaundice among successful cases: about *90%* [5]

Specificity

For diagnosing normal pancreas, excluding failed cannulations: greater than *95%* [13]
False positives for extrapancreatic lesions can occur
     If regenerating cirrhotic nodules in liver are misinterpreted as malignant disease
False positives can also occur
     If spasm or failure to cannulate common bile duct suggests obstruction

Percutaneous Transhepatic Cholangiography (PTC)

Defines anatomy of biliary tract
Precisely diagnoses and locates obstructive lesion
Particularly useful if percutaneous drainage is planned
Indicates the presence of additional hepatic biliary lesions
Low failure rate with duct dilatation

Drawbacks

Invasive, with known complications (5% with hemorrhage, sepsis, bile peritonitis; .2% mortality) [15]

Success rate decreases with nondilated ducts: greater than 90% with dilated ducts, 70% with nondilated ducts (range 25–75%) [14, 18]

Comments

Should be followed by antibiotic coverage

Requires normal clotting mechanisms

Requires many needle passes to obtain high success rate [14]

Sensitivity

For detecting the site of obstruction after satisfactorily visualizing bile ducts: *88–100%* [16, 20]

For diagnosing specific etiology: *86%* in one series [20]

For detecting pancreatic carcinoma: approaching *100%* [3]

False negatives can occur

> With failure to puncture duct (this finding would tend to support nondilatation)

Specificity

For showing normal pancreas as normal: *95%* [3]

False positives can occur

> With peripancreatic metastases thought to be pancreatic [3]

Computed Tomography (CT)

Visualizes all areas of the pancreas equally well

Detects bile duct dilatation with or without masses in the head of pancreas

Provides information about more than biliary tract: gallbladder, liver (fatty infiltration or metastatic tumor), porta hepatis, pancreas, adrenals, and retroperitoneum

Drawbacks

Rare complications; occasional contrast reactions and/or secondary renal failure, with serious reactions only 1 in 14,000 [2]

Results may be affected by surgical clips or barium

As with ultrasound, stones in common duct can be missed

Sensitivity

For detecting disease of any sort in pancreas: nearly *90%* [7]

For detecting pancreatic mass and correctly classifying it as benign or malignant: about *85%* [7]

For determining level or site of obstruction: nearly *90%* [1]

For detecting the cause of obstruction (tumor vs. stone or inflammatory process): about *70%* [1]

False negatives can occur

> For pancreatic disease: if lesions are very small or patient

has insufficient fat to outline pancreas
For the level and/or site of biliary obstruction: rarely, because of poor technique

Specificity

For detecting normal pancreas: about *85–90%* [7, 13]
False positives can occur
For detecting pancreatic masses: if pancreatitis is present but no carcinoma

Contributions of Magnetic Resonance Imaging [8, 11]

Distinguishes dilated bile ducts from portal veins
Shows pancreatic masses and determines their cystic or solid character; however, not superior to CT

References

1. Baron, R. L., Stanley, R. J., Lee, J. K. T., et al. A prospective comparison of the evaluation of biliary obstruction using computed tomography and ultrasonography. *Radiology* 145: 91, 1982.
2. Broderick, T. W. Contrast Material Reactions. In G. W. Friedland, Filly, R. and M. J. Goris. (Eds.). *Uroradiology*. New York: Churchill Livingstone, 1983.
3. Freeny, P. C., and Ball, T. J. Endoscopic retrograde cholangiopancreatography (ERCP) and percutaneous transhepatic cholangiography (PTC) in the evaluation of suspected pancreatic carcinoma: Diagnostic limitations and contemporary roles. *Cancer* 47:1666, 1981.
4. Gold, R. P., Casarella, W. J., Stern, G., et al. Transhepatic cholangiography: The radiologic method of choice in suspected obstructive jaundice. *Radiology* 133:39, 1979.
5. Gregg, J. A., and McDonald, D.G. Endoscopic retrograde cholangiopancreatography and gray-scale abdominal ultrasound in the diagnosis of jaundice. *Am. J. Surg.* 137:611, 1979.,
6. Gross, B. H., Harter, L. P., Gore, R. M., et al. Ultrasonic evaluation of common bile duct stones: Prospective comparison with endoscopic retrograde cholangiopancreatography. *Radiology* 146:471, 1983.
7. Hessel, S. J., Siegelman, S. S., McNeil, B. J., et al. A prospective evaluation of computed tomography and ultrasound of the pancreas. *Radiology* 143:129, 1982.
8. Higgins, C. B., Goldberg, H., Hricak, H., et al. Nuclear magnetic resonance imaging of vasculature of abdominal viscera: Normal and pathologic features. *AJR* 140:1217, 1983.
9. Honickman, S. P., Mueller, P. R., Wittenberg, J., et al. Ultrasound in obstructive jaundice: Prospective evaluation of site and cause. *Radiology* 147:511, 1983.
10. Kamin, P. D., Bernardino, M. E., Wallace, S., et al. Comparison of ultrasound and computed tomography in the detection of pancreatic malignancy. *Cancer* 46:2410, 1980.

11. Kressel, H. Y., Axel, L., Thickman, D., et al. NMR imaging of the abdomen at 0.12 T. Initial clinical experience with a resistive magnet. *AJR* 141:1179, 1983.
12. Laing, F. C., and Jeffrey, R. B., Jr. Choledocholithiasis and cystic duct obstruction: Difficult ultrasonographic diagnosis. *Radiology* 146:475, 1983.
13. Moss, A. A., Federle, M., Shapiro, H. A., et al. The combined use of computed tomography and endoscopic retrograde cholangiopancreatography in the assessment of suspected pancreatic neoplasm: A blind clinical evaluation. *Radiology* 134:159, 1980.
14. Mueller, P. R., Harbin, W. P., Ferrucci, J. T., Jr, et al. Fine-needle transhepatic cholangiography: Reflections after 450 cases. *AJR* 136:85, 1981.
15. Nebel, O. T., Silvis, S. E., Rogers, G., et al. Complications associated with endoscopic retrograde cholangiopancreatography: Results of the 1974 A/S/G/E survey. *Gastrointest. Endosc.* 22:34, 1975.
16. Raval, B., Lamki, N., and Bandali, K. Radiologic investigation of suspected extrahepatic biliary obstruction. *Canad. Med. Assoc. J.* 127:1191, 1982.
17. Sample, F. W., Sarti, D. A., Goldstein, L. I., et al. Gray-scale ultrasonography of the jaundiced patient. *Radiology* 128:719, 1978.
18. Scharschmidt, B. F., Goldberg, H. I., and Schmid, R. Approach to the patient with cholestatic jaundice. *N. Engl. J. Med.* 308:1515, 1983.
19. Taylor, K. J. W., and Rosenfield, A. T. Grey-scale ultrasonography in the differential diagnosis of jaundice. *Arch. Surg.* 112:820, 1977.
20. Vas, W., and Salem, S. Accuracy of sonography and transhepatic cholangiography in obstructive jaundice. *J. Canad. Assoc. Radiol.* 32:111, 1981.

5

Suspected Biliary Obstruction with Acute Pain

Robert A. Greenes and T. Edward Bynum

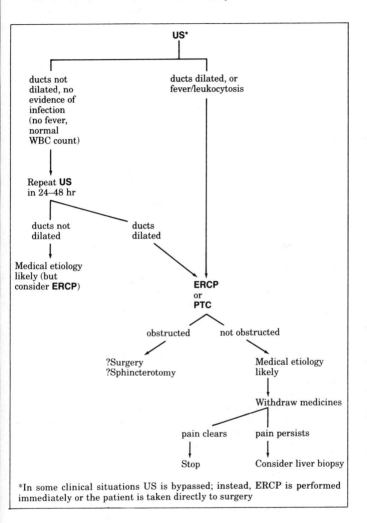

*In some clinical situations US is bypassed; instead, ERCP is performed immediately or the patient is taken directly to surgery

Typical Patient

Individual experiencing upper abdominal pain, often with gallstones, with or without clinical jaundice. An elevated bilirubin and an "obstructive" (cholestatic) chemical pattern are often present.

Typical Disorder(s)

Gallstones

Rarely, mechanical obstruction due to tumor or diseases related to hepatocellular dysfunction (e.g., acute hepatitis) or to intrahepatic cholestasis

Comment

Computed tomography is not needed or recommended in the clinical situation that the algorithm addresses except for extremely obese patients for whom ultrasound would be technically unsuccessful

Ultrasound (US)

Confirms an already high clinical suspicion of stones by either visualizing them directly or, more likely, by seeing dilated ducts

Defines size of common bile duct and intrahepatic biliary tract

Drawbacks

Except for masses in head of pancreas or (sometimes) calculi, seldom identifies the cause of obstruction

Excessive bowel gas, ascites, and obesity can affect results

In postcholecystectomy patients, ultrasound assessment of duct size correlates poorly with biliary disease

Sensitivity

For detecting obstruction (common duct more than 8 mm): *88%* [1, 4]

For detecting stones in the cystic or common duct: *25–30%* [4, 5]

For detecting level of obstruction: *50–60%* [1, 9]

False negatives can occur

With nonvisualization of distal common duct

In many patients in early stages of acute (even high grade) obstruction having bile ducts that appear normal

Specificity

About *90%* [1]

False positives can occur

With chronic dilatation (e.g., post common duct exploration) without obstruction

Endoscopic Retrograde Cholangiopancreatography (ERCP)

Provides both diagnosis and location

Delineates pathology precisely

Success rate is 80–90% and is not dependent on dilated ducts [3]

Visualizes pancreatic duct

Sphincterotomy can be performed if necessary

Drawbacks

Occasional complications (5%: pancreatitis, sepsis, instrument injury, aspiration pneumonitis; .1% mortality) [7]

Highly operator dependent

Sensitivity

For detecting dilated bile ducts in general: about *80%*; if dilated ducts are associated with stones, about *90%* [3]

For diagnosing specific cause of jaundice among successful cases: about *90%* [3]

Specificity

For ruling out obstruction in hepatocellular disease: approaching *100%* [3]

False positives can occur (rarely)

    If spasm or failure to cannulate common bile duct suggests obstruction

Percutaneous Transhepatic Cholangiography (PTC)

Defines anatomy of biliary tract and obstructive lesion

Precisely diagnoses and locates obstructing lesion

Particularly useful if percutaneous drainage planned

Indicates the presence of additional hepatic biliary lesions

Drawbacks

Invasive, with known complications (5%, with hemorrhage, sepsis, bile peritonitis; .2% mortality) [7]

Success rate decreases with nondilated ducts: greater than 90% with dilated ducts, 70% with nondilated ducts (range 25–75%) [6, 9]

Comments

Should be followed by antibiotic coverage

Requires normal clotting mechanisms

May require many needle passes to obtain high success rate [6]

Sensitivity

For detecting obstruction after satisfactorily visualizing bile ducts: extremely high, *88–100%* [8, 10]

For diagnosing specific etiology: somewhat lower, *86%* in one series [10]

False negatives can occur

    With failure to puncture duct, which suggests that ducts may not be dilated

Approaching *100%* [8]

References

1. Baron, R. L., Stanley, R. J., Lee, J. K. T., et al. A prospective comparison of the evalution of ultrasonography. *Radiology* 145: 91, 1982.
2. Gold, R. P., Casarella, W. J., Stern, G., et al. Transhepatic cholangiography: The radiological method of choice in suspected obstructive jaundice. *Radiology* 133:39, 1979.
3. Gregg, J. A., and McDonald, D. G. Endoscopic retrograde cholangiopancreatography and gray-scale abdominal ultrasound in the diagnosis of jaundice. *Am. J. Surg.* 137:611, 1979.
4. Gross, B. H., Harter, L. P., Gore, R. M., et al. Ultrasonic evaluation of common bile duct stones: Prospective comparison with endoscopic retrograde cholangiopancreatography. *Radiology* 146:471, 1983.
5. Laing, R. C., and Jeffrey, R. B., Jr. Choledocholithiasis and cystic duct obstruction: Difficult ultrasonographic diagnosis. *Radiology* 146:475, 1983.
6. Mueller, P. R., Harbin, W. P., Ferrucci, J. T., Jr. et al. Fine-needle transhepatic cholangiography: Reflections after 450 cases. *AJR.* 136:85, 1981.
7. Nebel, O. T., Silvis, S. E., Rogers, G., Complications associated with endoscopic retrograde cholangiopancreatography: Results of the 1974 A/S/G/E survey. *Gastrointest. Endosc.* 22:34, 1975.
8. Raval, B., Lamki, N., and Bandali, K. Radiologic investigation of suspected extrahepatic biliary obstruction. *Canad. Med. Assoc. J.* 127:1191, 1982.
9. Scharschmidt, B. F., Goldberg, H. I., and Schmid, R. Approach to the patient with cholestatic jaundice. *N. Engl. J. Med.* 308:1515, 1983.
10. Vas, W., and Salem, S. Accuracy of sonography and transhepatic cholangiography in obstructive jaundice. *J. Canad. Assoc. Radiol.* 32:111, 1981.

6

Acute Upper Gastrointestinal Bleeding

John M. Braver

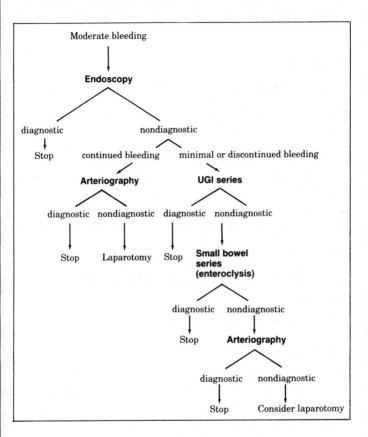

Typical Patient

Individual with hematemesis, bloody gastric aspirate, or melena thought to be related to upper gastrointestinal bleeding

Typical Disorder(s)

Esophageal ulcers or erosions
Gastric ulcers or erosions
Duodenal ulcers
Varices

Comments

Diagnostic approach depends on the clinical status: If bleeding is moderate and hemoglobin can be maintained, endoscopy and GI series may be undertaken; if bleeding is rapid, arteriography for localization and therapeutic purposes is indicated.

In some cases patients with moderate bleeding from an unknown cause may benefit from a labeled RBC study (see Chap. 7, p. 35) before arteriography

Endoscopy

Gold standard: Visual inspection indicates that lesion identified is the one actually bleeding

Frequently detects more bleeding lesions than does UGI series

Drawbacks

Rare perforations: 0.3 per 1,000 with .004% deaths overall [16]

Occasional hypotension secondary to premedications

Sometimes difficult or impossible in patients with esophageal strictures

Sensitivity

For identifying primary bleeding site: *80–95%* [4, 5, 13, 19]

False negatives can occur

In the presence of very rapid bleeding with large amounts of fresh blood and clots that obscure lesions

Specificity

For making specific diagnosis: greater than *95%* [4, 13]

Arteriography

Method of choice for acute rapid bleeding

Demonstrates lesions like angiodysplasia, not diagnosable on barium studies

Useful in localizing the bleeding site in duodenal and gastric lesions; usually does not demonstrate bleeding varices

Occasionally shows the characteristic vascular pattern of tumors in the small intestine not readily detected by barium study

Drawbacks

Complications: contrast reaction and/or secondary renal failure, rare; vascular injury and thrombosis, serious, about 1%; local hemorrhage or hematoma, nonfatal serious reactions, less than 2%; fatalities, .03% [9]

If volume of bleeding is less than 0.5 cc per minute at the time of injection, bleeding site is unlikely to be defined

Comment

Catheter is placed in celiac or superior mesenteric artery

Sensitivity

In detecting bleeding sites: *75–85%* [1, 2, 17]
False negatives can occur
> If bleeding stops just before or during examination or is less than 0.5 cc per minute

Specificity

High

Upper Gastrointestinal (UGI) Series

Indicated only when acute bleeding has been controlled and patient can undergo a procedure that may define nature of lesion and exact bleeding site
Relatively accurate in patients with peptic ulcer and varices

Drawbacks

Mucosal lesions may be frequently missed
Ulcers and carcinoma may be missed
Bleeding site cannot be defined with assurance in some patients
Retained barium in intestine may preclude satisfactory arteriography for 1 or 2 days if rebleeding occurs

Comments

With cessation of bleeding, procedure is a rational, noninvasive starting point
As an emergency procedure, accuracy is less than 50%

Sensitivity

For identifying primary bleeding site: quite variable, from *34–82%* [3, 6, 11, 13]
False negatives can occur
> If the size of lesion limits detectability

Specificity

For making specific diagnoses: lower than endoscopy, but, among all patients with UGI bleeding, fewer than 10% false positive diagnoses [4, 13]
False positives can occur
> If barium trapped between fold simulates ulcer collections

Small Bowel Series (Enteroclysis)

Demonstrates either jejunoileal ulcer or neoplasm
Best method of examining entire small intestine
Enteroclysis (tube injection near ligament of Treitz) is essential for adequate study
Fluoroscopy and films must be performed at intervals to avoid missing lesions
Instillation of methylcellulose affords a double contrast study

Drawbacks

Incomplete without fluoroscopy throughout examination

Sensitivity

No data available but sensitivity of small bowel follow-through is increased substantially by enteroclysis [12]: Up to 50% of patients will have more information provided

Specificity

No data available, but specificity of small bowel follow-through is obtained with enteroclysis

References

1. Baum, S., Nusbaum, M., Clearfield, H. R., et al. Angiography in the diagnosis of gastrointestinal bleeding. *Arch. Intern. Med.* 119:16, 1967.
2. Butler, M. L., Johnson, L. F., and Clark, R. Diagnostic accuracy of fiberoptic panendoscopy and visceral angiography in acute upper gastrointestinal bleeding. *Am. J. Gastroenterol.* 65:501, 1976.
3. Cello, J. P., and Thoeni, R. F. Gastrointestinal hemorrhage: Comparative values of double-contrast upper gastrointestinal radiology and endoscopy. *JAMA* 243:685, 1980.
4. Dooley, C. P., Larson, A. W., Stace, N. H., et al. Double-contrast barium meal and upper gastrointestinal endoscopy: A comparative study. *Ann. Intern. Med.* 101:538, 1984.
5. Dronfield, M. W., Langman, M. J. S., Atkinson, M., et al. Outcome of endoscopy and barium radiography for acute upper gastrointestinal bleeding: Controlled trial in 1037 patients. *Br. Med. J.* 284:545, 1982.
6. Dronfield, M. W., McIllmurray, M. B., Ferguson, R., et al. A prospective, randomized study of endoscopy and radiology in acute upper-gastrointestinal-tract bleeding. *Lancet* 1:1167, 1977.
7. Engelstad, B. L., and Hattner, R. S. New scintigraphic methods of detecting and localizing gastrointestinal bleeding. *Appl. Radiol.* July-August: 85, 1983.
8. Frey, C. F., Reuter, S. R., and Bookstein, J. J. Localization of gastrointestinal hemorrhage by selective angiography. *Surgery* 67:548, 1970.
9. Hessel, S. J. Complications of Angiography and Other Catheter Procedures. In H. L. Abrams (Ed.). *Abrams Angiography: Vascular and Interventional Radiology* (3rd ed.). Boston: Little, Brown, 1983. Pp. 1041–1055.
10. Katon, R. M., and Smith, F. W. Panendoscopy in the early diagnosis of acute upper gastrointestinal bleeding. *Gastroenterology* 65:728, 1973.
11. Keller, R. T., and Logan, G. M., Jr. Comparison of emergent endoscopy and upper gastrointestinal series radiography in acute upper gastrointestinal hemorrhage. *Gut* 17:180, 1976.
12. Maglinte, D. D. T., Burney, B. T., and Miller, R. E. Lesions missed on small-bowel follow-through: Analysis and recommendations. *Radiology* 144:737, 1982.

13. McGinn, F. P., Guyer, P. B., Wilken, B. J., et al. A prospective comparative trial between early endoscopy and radiology in acute upper gastrointestinal haemorrhage. *Gut* 16:707, 1975.
14. Rabe, F. E., Becker, G. J., Besozzi, M. J., et al. Efficacy study of the small-bowel examination. *Radiology* 140:47, 1981.
15. Schiller, K. F. R., Cotton, P. B., and Salmon, P. R. The hazards of digestive fibre-endoscopy. A survey of British experience. *Gut* 13:1027, 1982.
16. Silvis, S. E., Nebel, O., Rogers, G., et al. Endoscopic complications: Results of the 1974 American Society for Gastrointestinal Endoscopy survey. *JAMA* 235:928, 1976.
17. Stanley, R. J., and Wise, L. Arteriography in diagnosis of acute gastrointestinal tract bleeding. *Arch. Surg.* 107:138, 1973.
18. Steer, M., and Silen, W. Diagnostic procedures in gastrointestinal hemorrhage. *N. Engl. J. Med.* 309:646, 1983.
19. Zambartas, C., Cregeen, R. J., Forrest, J. A. H., et al. Accuracy of early endoscopy in acute upper gastrointestinal bleeding. *Br. Med. J.* 285:1540, 1982.

Acute Lower Gastrointestinal Bleeding

John M. Braver

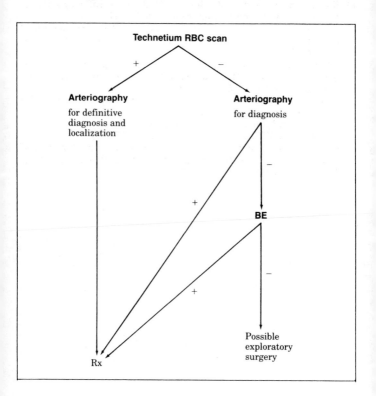

Typical Patient

Individual experiencing sudden onset of brisk rectal bleeding
  without blood in gastric aspirate

Typical Disorder(s)

Diverticulosis
Angiodysplasia
Ischemic colitis
Inflammatory bowel disease (rarely)

Comments

Hemorrhoids are the most common cause of lower gastrointestinal bleeding; history and proctoscopy will exclude their pres-

ence, and this algorithm assumes that proctoscopy has already been done

Carcinomas and polyps may cause acute lower gastrointestinal bleeding but more commonly are associated with chronic bleeding and are included under that algorithm (see Chap. 8)

Colonoscopy, valuable for chronic or subacute bleeding, is *not* the examination of choice for acute rapid bleeding; fresh blood and clots preclude a good view of mucosa [7, 9, 16]

Technetium Red Blood Cell (RBC) Scan

Confirms the presence of active bleeding as low as 0.1 ml per minute [1]

Localizes the approximate bleeding site as a guide for angiography

> If activity is detected soon after injection, there is a greater chance of accurately localizing the bleeding site

More sensitive than angiography, which requires active bleeding when contrast is injected

Labeled red blood cells are preferable to labeled sulfur colloid [4]

> They are more sensitive
>
> Because cells do not accumulate in the liver and spleen, there is better visualization of the upper abdomen above the ligament of Treitz
>
> Images can be repeated 24 hours later; active bleeding is not necessary at the time of injection

Drawbacks

Peristalsis moves labeled material from original site and can cause false positive localizations

Sensitivity

For detection: very high but difficult to quantify exactly

> In comparison to angiography: *80–90%* [12, 13, 19]

For detection and localization: very high

> One study localized *85%* of lower GI bleeds correctly [13]

Probability of a positive study increases with the number of transfusions; if more than one unit is required: *30%* [13]

False negatives can occur

> In the absence of active bleeding during imaging period

Comment

The number of false negatives decreases the longer the time period over which images are collected

Specificity

About *90%* [19]

False positives can occur

> If free pertechnetate is found in red blood cell preparation

Arteriography

Provides the most definitive diagnosis

May demonstrate underlying etiology of bleeding; shows lesions such as angiodysplasia (not diagnosable on barium enema); and may reveal vascular pattern of small intestine tumors not readily detected by barium

Essential for nonsurgical therapy

> With localized bleeding site, vasopressin infusion or injection of embolic material can stop bleeding

Bleeding site found in about 40% of those with acute lower GI bleeds [2, 14] and sometimes in as many as 53% [3] by using arteriography

Drawbacks

Complications: contrast reaction and/or secondary renal failure, rare; vascular injury and thrombosis, serious, about 1%; local hemorrhage or hematoma, nonfatal serious reactions, less than 2%; fatalities, .03% [10]

Rarely shows intraluminal contrast because of the relatively slow bleeding rate associated with chronic bleeding

Comments

Requires bleeding rate of about 0.5 ml per minute

Sensitivity

No data available for detecting bleeding; however, many patients will have a positive RBC scan, a bleeding site demonstrated surgically, and a negative arteriogram [20]

For localizing bleeding: No data, but a pressure injection into one part of the system may alter flow dynamics and suggest an inaccurate bleeding site

False negatives can occur if

> Bleeding has stopped completely
>
> Bleeding has stopped temporarily secondary to transient hypotension from vasovagal reaction or blood loss
>
> Incorrect vessel has been injected

Specificity

High

False positives are very rare, particularly in lower GI bleeds; however

> Superimposed renal calyx can cause false positives
>
> If lumbar artery is injected, normal blush can resemble extravasation

Barium Enema (BE)

Does not detect bleeding as such

Excellent for defining carcinoma and polyps when active bleeding has ceased

Demonstrates ischemia and inflammatory colitis well
Should be reserved for cases in which neither RBC scan nor an-
giography detects bleeding site
Should be performed when bleeding is controlled

Drawbacks

Not helpful in diagnosing angiodysplasia and bleeding divertic-
ula, the most common causes of acute rapid colonic bleeding
Bowel preparation needed
Rare possibility of perforation

Sensitivity

Sensitive for detecting carcinoma (*90%*) [6], polyps (*90%* of those
larger than 2 cm [15]), and colitis but incapable of detecting
bleeding per se

Specificity

No data available; however,
False positives can occur
    In the presence of fecal contamination

References

1. Alavi, A., Dann, R. W., Baum, S., et al. Scintigraphic detection of
   acute gastrointestinal bleeding. *Radiology* 124:753, 1977.
2. Bar, A. H., DeLaurentis, D. A., Parry, C. E., et al. Angiography in
   the management of massive lower gastrointestinal tract hemorrhage. *Surg. Gynecol. Obstet.* 150:226, 1980.
3. Baum, S. Angiography and the gastrointestinal bleeder. *Radiology* 143:569, 1982.
4. Bunker, S. R., Lull, R. J., Tanasescu, D. E., et al. Scintigraphy of
   gastrointestinal hemorrhage: Superiority of ^{99m}Tc red blood cells
   over ^{99m}Tc sulfur colloid. *AJR* 143:543, 1984.
5. Casarella, W. J., Galloway, S. J., Taxin, R. N., et al. "Lower" gastrointestinal tract hemorrhage: New concepts based on arteriography. *AJR* 121:357, 1974.
6. Cooley, R. N., Agnew, C. H., and Rios, G. Diagnostic accuracy of
   the barium enema study in carcinoma of the colon and rectum.
   AJR 84:316, 1960.
7. Gelfand, D. W., Wu, W. C., and Ott, D. J. The extent of successful
   colonoscopy: Its implication for the radiologist. *Gastrointest. Radiol.* 4:75, 1979.
8. Halpern, M. Percutaneous transfemoral arteriography: An analysis of the complications in 1,000 consecutive cases. *AJR* 92:918,
   1964.
9. Hedberg, S. E. Endoscopy in gastrointestinal bleeding. A system-
   atic approach to diagnosis. *Surg. Clin. North Am.* 54:549, 1974.
10. Hessel, S. J. Complications of Angiography and Other Catheter
    Procedures. In H. L. Abrams (Ed.). *Abrams Angiography: Vascu-
    lar and Interventional Radiology* (3rd ed.). Boston: Little, Brown,
    1983. Pp. 1041–1055.

11. Lang, E. K. A survey of the complications of percutaneous retrograde arteriography: Seldinger technic. *Radiology* 81:257, 1963.

12. Markisz, J. A., Front, D., Royal, H. D., et al. An evaluation of ^{99m}Tc-labeled red blood cell scintigraphy for the detection and localization of gastrointestinal bleeding sites. *Gastroenterology* 83:394, 1982.

13. McKusick, K. A., Froelich, J., Callahan, R. J., et al. [99m]Tc red blood cells for detection of gastrointestinal bleeding: Experience with 80 patients. *AJR* 137:1113, 1981.

14. Rahn, N. H., III, Tishler, J. M., Han, S. Y., et al. Diagnostic and interventional angiography in acute gastrointestinal hemorrhage. *Radiology* 143:361, 1982.

15. Raufmann, J. P., and Dobbins, W. O. Evaluation of Chronic Gastrointestinal Blood Loss. In R. G. Fiddian-Green and J. G. Turcotte (Eds.). *Gastrointestinal Hemorrhage.* New York: Grune & Stratton, 1980. Pp. 23–38.

16. Sivak, M. V., Jr., Sullivan, B. H., Jr., and Rankin, G. B. Colonoscopy: A report of 644 cases and review of the literature. *Am. J. Surg.* 128:351, 1974.

17. Thoeni, R. F., and Petras, A. Double-contrast barium-enema examination and endoscopy in the detection of polypoid lesions in the cecum and ascending colon. *Radiology* 144:257, 1982.

18. Thoeni, R. F., and Venbrux, A. C. The value of colonoscopy and double-contrast barium-enema examinations in the evaluation of patients with subacute and chronic lower intestinal bleeding. *Radiology* 146:603, 1983.

19. Winzelberg, G. G., Froelich, J. W., McKusick, K. A., et al. Radionuclide localization of lower gastrointestinal hemorrhage. *Radiology* 139:465, 1981.

20. Winzelberg, G. G., McKusick, K. A., Froelich, J. W., et al. Detection of gastrointestinal bleeding with ^{99m}Tc-labeled red blood cells. *Semin. Nucl. Med.* 12:139, 1982.

8

Chronic Gastrointestinal Bleeding

John M. Braver

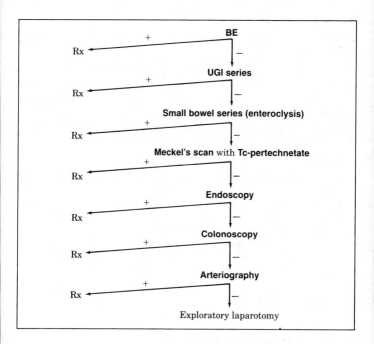

Typical Patient

Individual with low-grade bleeding in association with anemia, confirmed by stool guaiac or low hematocrit

Typical Disorder(s)

Polyps
Cancer
Ulcers, gastritis
Meckel's diverticulum
Angiodysplasia
Benign intramural neoplasms

Barium Enema (BE)

Highly accurate for polyps and cancer
Excellent demonstration of chronic inflammatory lesions
When skillfully performed, air contrast studies elegantly demonstrate mucosal detail

Reflux through the ileocecal valve permits an excellent view of the terminal ilium, for most patients

With negative test results, barium evacuation permits upper gastrointestinal examination

Drawbacks

Uncomfortable; difficult for those with low tolerance or with inflammatory disease

High pressure in the colon in acute inflammatory disease is sometimes associated with perforation

Without a clean colonic mucosa, the examination is inaccurate and the distinction between polyps and fecal material is difficult

A standard barium enema without air contrast can miss 40% of polypoid lesions and 20% of carcinomas [8]

Sensitivity

For all causes of subacute and chronic bleeds in general: *70%* [14]

For polyps and compared to colonoscopy: *27%* for polyps less than 1 cm; *83%* for polyps between 1 and 2 cm; and greater than *90%* for polyps more than 2 cm [8]

For bleeding polyps in these patients: greater than *90%* [14]

High for most cancers (*80–85%*), but lower for low-lying rectal carcinomas where sigmoidoscopy is better

Specificity

About 10% of lesions thought to be carcinoma are not [6]

Upper Gastrointestinal (UGI) Series

Simple and accurate for esophagogastric polyps, carcinoma, peptic ulcer, and large esophageal varices

Gastric air contrast studies, although more complex, are useful for small mucosal tumors

Drawbacks

Barium remaining in the intestine precludes other examinations (arteriography, for example) for 1 to 2 days

Sensitivity

For detecting duodenal ulcers using double contrast examinations: about 80–90% [6]; using single contrast technique, only *70–80%* of ulcers visualized on endoscopy are seen [6]

Specificity

Very high

False positives can occur

    If small diverticulum is thought to be an ulcer crater

    If barium trapped between fold simulates ulcer collections

Small Bowel Series (Enteroclysis)

See features, drawbacks, and comments listed in Chapter 6, p. 31

Comments

In this context the examination is performed primarily to detect intramural neoplasms or chronic inflammatory disease

Sensitivity

Enteroclysis has a higher sensitivity than conventional small bowel follow-through; the yield of the latter among all patients with subacute or chronic bleeding is very low, about 5% [3, 7]; when specific small bowel pathology is suspected, yield is higher, about 50% [3]

Specificity

Enteroclysis has a higher specificity than small bowel follow-through; in both cases, however, there are very few false positives if a bona fide filling defect or characteristic inflammatory lesions are seen

Meckel's Scan (Tc-Pertechnetate)

Pertechnetate concentrates in the gastric mucosa of the Meckel's diverticulum

Comments

Relatively low yield because of the rarity of the Meckel's diverticulum, especially in adults
Probably should be the last noninvasive examination performed because of low yield

Sensitivity

Overall: 85% [10]; sensitivity may increase if provocative agents (e.g., histamine) are used
False negatives can occur
    If the diverticulum contains mucosa other than gastric
    If gastric mucosa is insufficient in mass or function
    With dilution and wash away by hemorrhage
    With overlapping organs (bladder, duodenum)

Specificity

Overall: 95% [10]
False positives can occur in the presence of
    Inflammatory lesions
    Arteriovenous malformations
    Ulcers
    Some bowel tumors
    Urinary tract abnormalities

Endoscopy

See features, drawbacks, and comments listed in Chapter 6,
 p. 30

Comments

In this context examination is performed primarily to detect ulcer, gastritis, or neoplasm

Sensitivity

For detecting duodenal ulcers: *90–100%* [6]
Will detect at least 5% more lesions than seen on air contrast
 upper GI series [8]

Specificity

Very high, but false positives for gastritis can occur if anteced-
 ent lavage is too vigorous

Colonoscopy

When skillfully performed, highly accurate for defining colonic
 pathology
Complements barium enema; will find the cause of bleeding in
 40% of patients with negative radiographic studies and negative sigmoidoscopies

Drawbacks

Requires preparation: liquid diet for 2 days and enemas
Contraindicated in uncooperative patients or those with acute
 myocardial infarctions
Complications: morbidity, particularly hemorrhage, 0.5–1.3%;
 mortality, .02% [6]

Sensitivity

For all causes of subacute and chronic bleeds: greater than
 90% [14]

Arteriography

Demonstrates lesions such as angiodysplasia, which can rarely
 be diagnosed on barium studies
Can reveal the characteristic vascular patterns of tumors in the
 small intestine not detected by barium studies

Drawbacks

Complications: contrast reaction and/or secondary renal failure,
 rare; vascular injury and thrombosis, serious, about 1%; local
 hemorrhage or hematoma, nonfatal serious reactions, less
 than 2%; fatalities, .03% [4]

Comment

Rarely shows intraluminal bleeding because of the relatively slow rate of bleeding

Sensitivity

May be as high as *45%* for patients with subacute or chronic bleeding. Of these, more than 50% will have vascular malformations or visceral artery aneurysms; the rest will be miscellaneous causes, such as carcinoma, polyps, Meckel's diverticulum [11].

False negatives can occur in the presence of
Meckel's diverticulum, carcinoma, leiomyoma, Crohn's disease, phlebectasia

Specificity

Approaching *100%* [11]

References

1. Best, E. B., Teaford, A. K., and Rader, F. H., Jr. Angiography in chronic/recurrent gastrointestinal bleeding: A nine-year study. *Surg. Clin. North Am.* 59:811, 1979.
2. Conway, J. J., and the Pediatric Nuclear Club of the Society of Nuclear Medicine. The sensitivity, specificity and accuracy of radionuclide imaging of Meckel's diverticulum (abstract). *J. Nucl. Med.* 17:553, 1976.
3. Fried, A. M., Poulos, A., and Hatfield, D. R. The effectiveness of the incidental small-bowel series. *Radiology* 140:45, 1981.
4. Hessel, S. J. Complications of Angiography and Other Catheter Procedures. In H. L. Abrams (Ed.). *Abrams Angiography: Vascular and Interventional Radiology* (3rd ed.). Boston: Little, Brown, 1983. Pp. 1041–1055.
5. Hogan, W. J., Stewart, E. T., Geenen, J. E., et al. A prospective comparison of the accuracy of colonoscopy vs. barium contrast exam for detection of colonic polypoid lesions. *Gastrointest. Endosc.* 23:230, 1977.
6. McGuigan, J. L. Peptic Ulcer. In *Harrison's Principles of Internal Medicine* (10th ed.). New York: McGraw-Hill, 1983.
7. Rabe, F. E., Becker, G. J., Besozzi, M. J. et al. Efficacy study of the small-bowel examination. *Radiology* 140; 47, 1981.
8. Raufmann, J.-P., and Dobbins, W. O., III. Evaluation of Chronic Gastrointestinal Blood Loss. In R. G. Fiddian-Green and J. G. Turcotte (Eds.). *Gastrointestinal Hemorrhage.* New York: Grune & Stratton, 1980. Pp. 23–38.
9. Rosenthall, L., Henry, J. N., Murphy, D. A., et al. Radiopertechnetate imaging of the Meckel's diverticulum. *Radiology* 105:371, 1972.
10. Sfakinakis, G. N., and Conway, J. J. Detection of ectopic gastric mucosa in Meckel's diverticulum and in other aberrations by scintigraphy. ii. Indications and methods—a 10-year experience. *J. Nucl. Med.* 22:732, 1981.

11. Sheedy, P. F., II, Fulton, R. E., and Atwell, D. T. Angiographic evaluation of patients with chronic gastrointestinal bleeding. *AJR* 123:338, 1975.
12. Steer, M. L., and Silen, W. Diagnostic procedures in gastrointestinal hemorrhage. *N. Engl. J. Med.* 309:646, 1983.
13. Stroehlein, J. R., Goulston, K., and Hunt, R. H. Diagnostic approach to evaluating the cause of a positive fecal occult blood test. *CA—A Cancer Journal for Clinicians* 34:148, 1984.
14. Thoeni, R. F., and Venbrux, A. C. The value of colonoscopy and double-contrast barium-enema examinations in the evaluation of patients with subacute and chronic lower intestinal bleeding. *Radiology* 146:603, 1983.

9

Palpable Abdominal Mass

Robert P. Fortunato

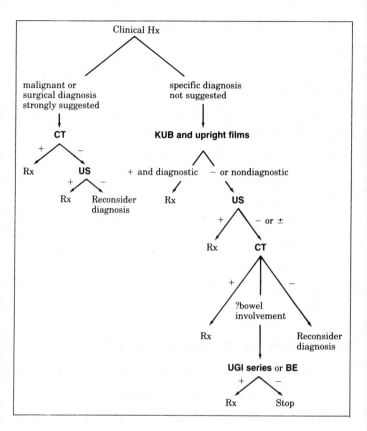

Typical Patient

Individual experiencing abdominal distress who has observed
abdominal swelling or felt a mass, or whose physician has pal-
pated a mass; sometimes felt on routine physical examination
in asymptomatic individuals

Typical Disorder(s)

The range of abnormalities covered in this algorithm is large. In
one study [4] typical final pathological diagnoses in patients
with palpable abdominal masses were:

	%
No abnormality	14
Ovarian mass	23

Liver enlargement, liver tumor, or diseased gallbladder	17
Kidney enlargement, mass	13
Pancreas enlargement or tumor	6
Aortic aneurysm	25
Miscellaneous masses or fluid collections	2

Comments

Examinations for palpable abdominal mass have the same general features and drawbacks as those described in Chapter 1. Please note the following comments.

In this clinical setting one study [4] indicated that ultrasound's accuracy was more than 95%, hence its prominent place in the algorithm; however, there were problems in identifying the origins of large lesions

One randomized study [1] showed CT to be the most cost-effective approach for evaluation, with sensitivity approaching 100% for detecting abnormalities and a slightly lower value for definitive diagnosis; specificity also approached 100%

  Other radiographic modalities were slightly less sensitive for detection and diagnosis and were also slightly less specific

When abdominal mass occurs in a patient with preexisting cancer (e.g., of bowel), laparoscopy or laparotomy may be necessary even in the face of normal CT and ultrasound examinations; both examinations may be falsely negative in the retroperitoneum, particularly after an abdominoperineal resection

Contribution of Magnetic Resonance Imaging [3, 5]

Demonstrates abdominal and retroperitoneal vascular anatomy without IV contrast

Plays a similar role to CT in identifying location, size, and origin of masses

Whether MRI augments CT and other methods' capacity to identify the nature of a mass is as yet uncertain

References

1. Dixon, A. K., Fry, I. K., Kingham, J. G. C., et al. Computed tomography in patients with an abdominal mass: Effective and efficient? A controlled trial. *Lancet* 1:1199, 1981.
2. Hessel, S. J., Siegelman, S. S., McNeil, B. J., et al. A prospective evaluation of computed tomography and ultrasound of the pancreas. *Radiology* 143:129, 1982.
3. Higgins, C. B., Goldberg, H., Hricak, H., et al. Nuclear magnetic resonance imaging of vasculature of abdominal viscera: Normal and pathologic features. *AJR* 140:1217, 1983.

4. Holm, H. H., Gammelgaard, J., Jensen, F., et al. Ultrasound in the diagnosis of a palpable abdominal mass: A prospective study of 107 patients. *Gastrointest. Radiol.* 7:149, 1982.
5. Lee, J. K. T., Heiken, J. P., Ling, D., et al. Magnetic resonance imaging of abdominal and pelvic lymphadenopathy. *Radiology* 153:181, 1984.
6. Lee, J. K. T., Stanley, R. J., Melson, G. L., et al. Pancreatic imaging by ultrasound and computed tomography. *Radiol. Clin. North Am.* 16:105, 1979.
7. Sanders, R. C., McNeil, B. J., Finberg, H. J., et al. A prospective study of computed tomography and ultrasound in the detection and staging of pelvic masses. *Radiology* 146:439, 1983.

10

Suspected Renal Mass

Peter M. Doubilet and Steven E. Seltzer

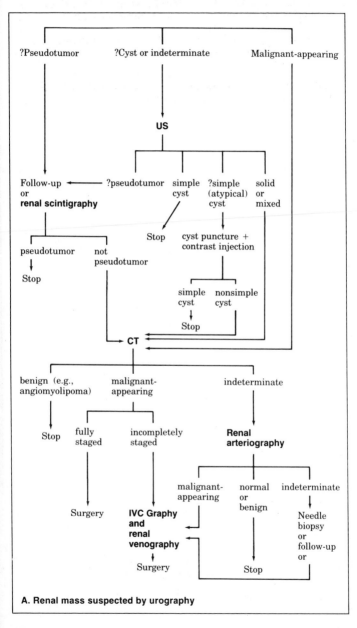

A. Renal mass suspected by urography

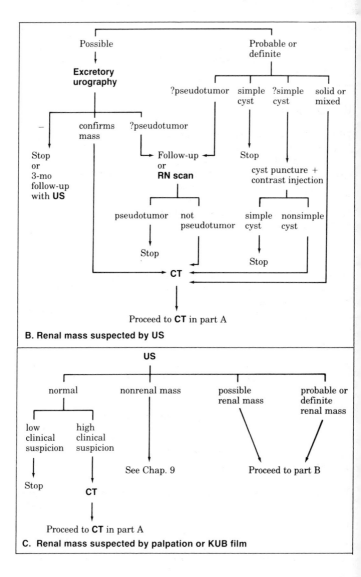

B. Renal mass suspected by US

C. Renal mass suspected by palpation or KUB film

Typical Patient

Individual with renal mass suspected on the basis of excretory urogram, ultrasound, palpation, or KUB

Typical Disorder(s)

Renal neoplasms and cysts
Column of Bertin

Comment

In this situation the issue is not identifying a mass but, in most cases, confirming its presence or differentiating a benign cyst from a tumor

Ultrasound (US)

Differentiates cyst from solid mass
Demonstrates caval involvement
Detects nonrenal lesions
Provides presumptive diagnosis of angiomyolipoma

Drawbacks

Obesity can cause poor visualization
Excessive gas can affect results

Sensitivity

For differentiating cysts from tumors: very high; *84–98%* of neo-plasms will be correctly identified as such when a mass thought to be either a cyst or tumor is present [2, 5, 10]
False negatives can occur
  With cystic or necrotic lesions having small focal area(s) of neoplastic tissue in the wall

Specificity

Very high: *88–100%* of cysts will be correctly identified as such when a mass thought to be either a cyst or tumor is present [2, 5, 10]
False positives can occur
  If artifacts cause internal echoes in simple cysts

Renal Scintigraphy Using ^{99}Tc-DMSA or ^{99m}Tc-Glucoheptonate

Distinguishes pseudotumor, column of Bertin from renal mass
Defines renal masses, but not as precisely as ultrasound and CT

Drawbacks

Resolution not comparable with CT and ultrasound
Time of examination longer than with ultrasound

Sensitivity

High: *89%* of masses will be correctly identified as masses [9]

Specificity

High: *81%* of pseudotumors will be correctly identified as pseudotumors [9]

Computed Tomography (CT)

Differentiates cyst from tumor
Essential for staging of neoplasm
Defines inferior vena cava (IVC) accurately and renal vein involvement somewhat less accurately
Permits precise evaluation of contralateral kidney

Drawbacks

Possible contrast reactions

Sensitivity

Very high: nearly *100%* of solid masses [8] will be correctly identified as such when a mass thought to be either a cyst or tumor is present
In staging renal cell carcinoma [7, 11–13]
  For detecting perinephric extension: *83–100%*
  For detecting lymph node involvement: *73–90%*
  For detecting renal vein involvement: *50–86%*
  For detecting IVC extension: *75–100%*
  For detecting liver involvement: *67%*

Specificity

Very high: more than *98%* of cystic masses will be correctly identified as such when a mass thought to be either a cyst or tumor is present [8]
For staging renal cell carcinoma [7, 11–13] CT correctly shows no disease in
  Perinephric area: *75–100%*
  Lymph nodes: *81–100%*
  Renal vein: *84–100%*
  IVC: *92–100%*
  Liver: *100%*

Angiography (Renal Arteriography, Inferior Vena Cavography, Renal Venography)

Provides staging and diagnostic information with excellent detail of vascular anatomy and tumor extension into renal vein and inferior vena cava
Identifies renal cell carcinoma unequivocally when classical tumor vascular bed is defined

Drawbacks

Uncomfortable, with hospitalization generally required
Possible contrast reactions
Possible hematoma or thrombosis at catheter insertion site
Possible embolization or arterial dissection

Sensitivity

In staging renal cell carcinoma [7, 11–13]
>   For detecting perinephric extension: *59–93%*
>   For detecting lymph node involvement: *73–90%*
>   For detecting renal vein involvement: *75–100%*
>   For detecting IVC extension: *100%*
>   For detecting liver involvement: high

Specificity

For staging renal cell carcinoma [7, 11–13] angiography correctly shows no disease in
>   Perinephric area: *74–100%*
>   Lymph nodes: *81–100%*
>   Renal vein: *80–97%*
>   IVC: *100%*
>   Liver: high

Excretory Urography

May be useful follow-up to ultrasound that is mildly suspicious
for renal mass
An alternative, noninvasive method of imaging the kidneys

Drawbacks

Rare complications; occasional contrast reactions and/or secondary renal failure occur, with serious reactions only 1 in
14,000 [1]

Comments

Satisfactory renal function is required, although if higher contrast doses are used (which increase the risk of nephrotoxicity), some information can be produced in patients with poor
renal function

Sensitivity

Relatively high for renal masses; case reports of masses missed
by examination have been published [4], but no prospective
study to determine sensitivity has been published
False negatives can occur
>   From poor intestinal preparation
>   From technically poor examination or an imprecise exami-
>   nation protocol

Specificity

No precise data available, but high
False positives can occur
>   If normal variant (column of Bertin) is thought to be an ab-
>   normal mass

Contribution of Magnetic Resonance Imaging [3, 6]

Like CT, distinguishes cyst from neoplasm and abscess, and probably plays a role similar to CT in staging

Demonstrates the extension of tumors into the renal vein or inferior vena cava

References

1. Broderick, T. W. Contrast Material Reactions. In G. W. Friedland, R. Filly, and M. L. Goris (Eds.). *Uroradiology.* New York: Churchill Livingstone, 1983.
2. Clayman, R. V., Surya, V., Miller, R. P., et al. Pursuit of the renal mass: Is ultrasound enough? *Am. J. Med.* 77:218, 1984.
3. Hricak, H., Demas, B. E., Williams, R. D., et al. Magnetic resonance imaging in the diagnosis and staging of renal and perirenal neoplasms. *Radiology* 154:709, 1985.
4. Kass, D. A., Hricak, H., and Davidson, A. J. Renal malignancies with normal excretory urograms. *AJR* 141:731, 1983.
5. Leopold, G. R., Talner, L. B., Asher, W. M., et al. Renal ultrasonography: An updated approach to the diagnosis of renal cyst. *Radiology* 109:671, 1973.
6. Leung, A. W. L., Bydder, G. M., Steiner, R. E., et al. Magnetic resonance imaging of the kidneys. *AJR* 143:1215, 1984.
7. Love, L., Churchill, R., Reynes, C., et al. Computed tomography staging of renal carcinoma. *Urol. Radiol.* 1:3, 1979.
8. Magilner, A. D., and Ostrum, B. J. Computed tomography in the diagnosis of renal masses. *Radiology* 126:715, 1978.
9. Older, R. A., Korobkin, M., Workman, J., et al. Accuracy of radionuclide imaging in distinguishing renal masses from normal variants. *Radiology* 136:443, 1980.
10. Pollack, H. M., Banner, M. P., Arger, P. H., et al. The accuracy of gray-scale renal ultrasonography in differentiating cystic neoplasms from benign cysts. *Radiology* 143:741, 1982.
11. Probst, P., Hoogewoud, H. M., Haertel, M., et al. Computerized tomography versus angiography in the staging of malignant renal neoplasm. *Br. J. Radiol.* 54:744, 1981.
12. Richie, J. P., Garnick, M. B., Seltzer, S., et al. Computerized tomography scan for diagnosis and staging of renal cell carcinoma. *J. Urol.* 129:1114, 1983.
13. Weyman, P. J., McClennan, B. L., Stanley, R. J., et al. Comparison of computed tomography and angiography in the evaluation of renal cell carcinoma. *Radiology* 137:417, 1980.

Detection of Complications of Pancreatitis

Steven E. Seltzer

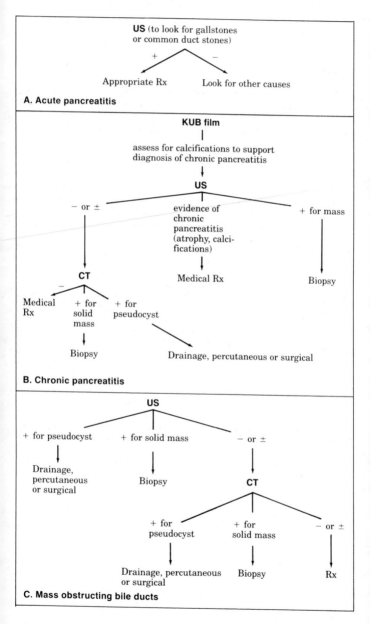

US (to look for gallstones or common duct stones)

\+ → Appropriate Rx

− → Look for other causes

A. Acute pancreatitis

KUB film

assess for calcifications to support diagnosis of chronic pancreatitis

US

− or ± → **CT**

− → Medical Rx

\+ for solid mass → Biopsy

\+ for pseudocyst → Drainage, percutaneous or surgical

evidence of chronic pancreatitis (atrophy, calcifications) → Medical Rx

\+ for mass → Biopsy

B. Chronic pancreatitis

US

\+ for pseudocyst → Drainage, percutaneous or surgical

\+ for solid mass → Biopsy

− or ± → **CT**

\+ for pseudocyst → Drainage, percutaneous or surgical

\+ for solid mass → Biopsy

− or ± → Rx

C. Mass obstructing bile ducts

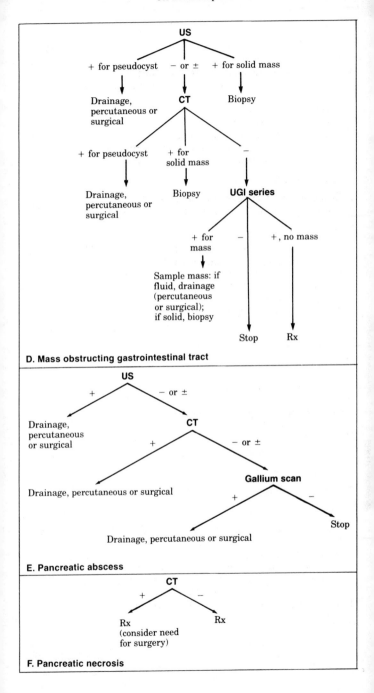

D. Mass obstructing gastrointestinal tract

E. Pancreatic abscess

F. Pancreatic necrosis

Typical Patient

Individual with acute midabdominal pain and biochemical evidence of pancreatitis

Individual who has had pancreatitis and who

Experiences persisting or increasing midabdominal pain and fever

Develops jaundice

Becomes nauseous, vomits

Experiences severe midabdominal pain along with fever and/or threatened cardiovascular collapse

Individual with chronic midabdominal pain

Typical Disorder(s)

Inflammatory disease of the pancreas

Inflammatory disease coexisting with carcinoma

Comments

If bile ducts are thought to be obstructed but CT and US are both either negative or equivocal (see algorithm, part C), then percutaneous transhepatic cholangiography may be indicated (see Chap. 5, p. 27, for a discussion of this technique under other circumstances).

ERCP is relatively contraindicated in patients with pancreatitis.

Ultrasound (US)

Rapid screening method

Available in any plane

Demonstrates mass lesions, but not with the accuracy of CT

Drawbacks

Quality of examination is impaired by gas, obesity, or barium

Comment

Morphological data are not so definitive as those of CT

Sensitivity

In acute pancreatitis excluding nondiagnostic examinations (about 40%): *38%* [15]

For pancreatic abscess detection, excluding nondiagnostic examinations (usually about 40%): *31–45%* [19]

For pseudocyst detection, excluding nondiagnostic examinations (about 40%): *87%* [5, 17]

For chronic pancreatitis, with high clinical suspicion: *33%* [4]

Specificity

For showing normal pancreas in patient suspected of pseudocyst, excluding nondiagnostic examinations (about 40%): *90%* [2, 17]

Computed Tomography (CT)

Method of choice to demonstrate pancreas
Defines adjacent tissues and organs well
Excellent demonstration of gross morphological characteristics

Comments

Requires both oral and intravenous contrast media for optimal
  results
Rare complications; occasional contrast reactions and/or secondary renal failure occur, but serious reactions only 1 in
  14,000 [3]

Sensitivity

For acute pancreatitis: *70%* [15]
For pancreatic abscess: *50%* [19]
For pseudocyst: *92%* [11, 17]
For chronic pancreatitis, with high clinical suspicion: *56%* [4]

Specificity

For showing normal pancreas in patients suspected of pseudocyst: *93%* [17]

Upper Gastrointestinal (UGI) Series

Useful in pinpointing the site and/or cause of mechanical bowel
  obstruction for this group of patients

Comments

Will only indirectly show a lesion arising from the pancreas or
  biliary tract
Should be performed after CT—otherwise barium will cause artifacts on CT

Sensitivity

No data available for UGI Series in this particular setting

Specificity

No data available for UGI Series in this particular setting

Gallium Scan

Detects infections/inflammations
Views the entire abdomen including bony structures

Drawbacks

Requires a 24- to 72-hour time delay for diagnosis
Results can be affected by intestinal activity, particularly during
  early examination

Recent surgical scar can show gallium activity for weeks, which can possibly interfere with interpretation

Unless imaging is done on Anger camera instead of rectilinear scanner, the sensitivity and specificity of the examination decrease significantly

Sensitivity

No data available specific for pancreatic disease, but very high; for detecting abdominal abscesses: lower than CT and higher than ultrasound, with range of reported values, probably about *80–90%* [6, 9, 10, 12]

False negatives can occur

In infections of very short duration

Specificity

No data available specific for pancreatic disease, but lower than CT, about *85%* [6, 10, 13] with some saying as low as *65%* [12] or as high as *95%* [9]

False positives can occur

Because of colonic activity, accumulation in coexisting tumors, in recent surgical wounds, and in inflammatory bowel disease

Contribution of Magnetic Resonance Imaging [1]

Delineates increased size and altered character of pancreas

Whether MRI can provide information beyond that afforded by CT is uncertain

References

1. Anacker, H., Rupp, N., and Reiser, M. Magnetic resonance (MR) in the diagnosis of pancreatic disease. *Eur. J. Radiol.* 4:265, 1984.
2. Andersen, B. N., Hancke, S., Nielsen, S. A. D., et al. The diagnosis of pancreatic cyst by endoscopic retrograde pancreatography and ultrasonic scanning. *Ann. Surg.* 185:286, 1977.
3. Broderick, T. W. Contrast Material Reactions. In G. W. Friedland, R. Filly, and M. L. Goris (Eds.). *Uroradiology.* New York: Churchill Livingstone, 1983.
4. Ferrucci, J. T., Wittenberg, J., Black, E. B., et al. Computed body tomography in chronic pancreatitis. *Radiology* 130:175, 1979.
5. Gonzalez, A. C., Bradley, E. L., and Clements, J. L., Jr. Pseudocyst formation in acute pancreatitis: Ultrasonographic evaluation of 99 cases. *AJR* 127:315, 1976.
6. Henkin, R. E. Gallium 67 in the Diagnosis of Inflammatory Disease. In P. B. Hoffer, C. Bekerman, and R. E. Henkin (Eds.). *Gallium-67 Imaging.* New York: Wiley, 1978. Pp. 65–83, 90–92.
7. Hessel, S. J., Siegelman, S. S., McNeil, B. J., et al. A prospective evaluation of computed tomography and ultrasound of the pancreas. *Radiology* 143:129, 1982.

8. Isikoff, M. B., Hill, M. C., Silverstein, W., et al. The clinical significance of acute pancreatic hemorrhage. *AJR* 136:679, 1981.

9. Kaplan, W. D. Imaging of Inflammatory Lesions. In P. B. Schneider and S. Treves (Eds.). *Nuclear Medicine in Clinical Practice.* North Holland: Elsevier, 1978. Pp. 299–310.

10. Korobkin, M., Callen, P. W., Filly, R. A., et al. Comparison of computed tomography, ultrasonography and gallium-67 scanning in the evaluation of suspected abdominal abscess. *Radiology* 129:89, 1978.

11. Kressel, H. Y., Margulis, A. R., Gooding, G. W., et al. CT scanning and ultrasound in the evaluation of pancreatic pseudocysts: A preliminary comparison. *Radiology* 126:153, 1978.

12. Moir, C., and Robins, R. E. Role of ultrasonography, gallium scanning and computed tomography in the diagnosis of intra-abdominal abscess. *Am. J. Surg.* 143:582, 1982.

13. Sfakianakis, G. N., Al-Sheikh, W., Heal, A., et al. Comparisons of scintigraphy with In-111 leukocytes and Ga-67 in the diagnosis of occult sepsis. *J. Nucl. Med.* 23:618, 1982.

14. Siegelman, S. S., Copeland, B. E., Saba, G. P., et al. CT of fluid collections associated with pancreatitis. *AJR* 134:1121, 1980.

15. Silverstein, W., Isikoff, M. B., Hill, M. C., et al. Diagnostic imaging of acute pancreatitis: Prospective study using CT and sonography. *AJR* 137:497, 1981.

16. Stanley, R. J., Sagel, S. S., and Levitt, R. G. Computed tomographic evaluation of the pancreas. *Radiology* 124:715, 1977.

17. Williford, M. E., Foster, W. L., Jr., Halvorsen, R. A., et al. Pancreatic pseudocyst: Comparative evaluation of sonography and computed tomography. *AJR* 140:53, 1983.

18. Wolfson, P. Surgical management of inflammatory disorders of the pancreas. *Surg. Gynecol. Obstet.* 151:689, 1980.

19. Woodard, S., Kelvin, F. M., Rice, R. P., et al. Pancreatic abscess: Importance of conventional radiology. *AJR* 136:871, 1981.

Blunt Abdominal Trauma

Sabah S. Tumeh

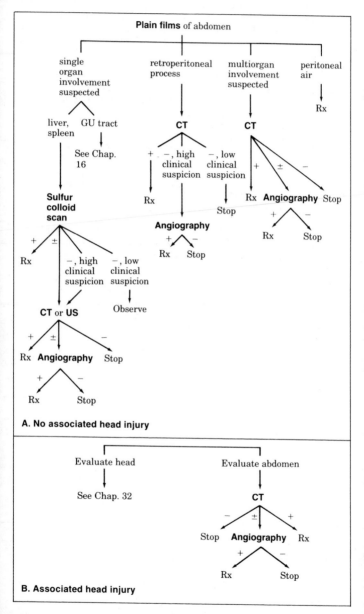

A. No associated head injury

B. Associated head injury

Typical Patient

Individual suspected of having an injury to the abdominal viscera after experiencing blunt trauma

Typical Disorder(s)

Acute vascular or parenchymal injuries in the abdomen

Computed Tomography (CT)

Provides simultaneous multiorgan visualization; about 10% of patients will have a clinically significant lesion outside of liver and spleen [7]

Evaluates presence of intraperitoneal fluid

Drawbacks

May require oral and rectal contrast; if patient is vomiting, however, oral contrast cannot be given

Rare complications; occasional contrast reactions and/or secondary renal failure occur, with serious reactions only 1 in 14,000 [2]

Metallic clips in abdomen (especially in upper abdomen) can reduce accuracy

Sensitivity

For detecting liver injuries: very high (no specific data)

For detecting splenic injuries: greater than 95% [3, 7]

For detecting intra- or retroperitoneal hematoma: very high

False negatives can occur

    From artifacts created by motion or clips

Specificity

For showing normal liver: very high

For showing normal spleen: 96% [7]

For showing normal retroperitoneum: very high

False positives can occur

    From artifacts created by motion or clips

    With inhomogeneous enhancement of spleen

Sulfur Colloid Scan

Determines site of injury in liver or spleen (particularly helpful for posterior superior quadrant of liver)

Detects concomitant active intraperitoneal bleed

Useful as baseline and then as means of monitoring repair, especially in spleen; defects should decrease—an enlarging defect is usually associated with expanding hematoma or posttraumatic cyst [4]

Drawbacks

Does not provide information about other organs (simultaneous injection of other radiotracer is occasionally used, however, to evaluate possibility of renal trauma)

Comment

If necessary, examination can be performed with a portable camera at bedside

Sensitivity

For detecting liver injuries: approaching *100%* [5, 9]
For detecting splenic injuries: *98%* [5, 9]
False negatives can occur
>   With very small lesions
>   With technically inadequate studies, i.e., an inadequate number of views in different obliquities

Specificity

For showing normal liver: *98%* [5]
For showing normal spleen: *96%* [5]
False positives can occur
>   In the presence of fetal lobulation and clefting with accessory spleens
>   From prior splenic trauma

Angiography

Accurately identifies presence and location of visceral or vascular injury
Provides a vascular road map for surgery, if required
Useful for nonoperative intervention to control bleeding

Drawbacks

Complications: contrast reaction and/or secondary renal failure, rare; vascular injury and thrombosis, serious, about 1%; local hemorrhage or hematoma, nonfatal serious reactions, less than 2%; fatalities, .03% [6]

Sensitivity

For detecting liver injuries: greater than *90%* [1, 8]
For detecting splenic injuries: greater than *90%* [1, 8]

Specificity

No precise data available, but presumably very high
False positives can occur in
>   Infarcts
>   Cysts
>   Lobulation

Ultrasound (US)

Defines large fluid collections well
Especially useful for pregnant women

Drawbacks

Cannot always be performed, e.g., if patient is in pain (19% in
one study [4])
Bowel gas, very common in patients with trauma, can possibly
lead to a technically unsatisfactory examination

Sensitivity

No data available but presumably high
False negatives can occur
    If examination is inadequate due to pain or bowel gas

Specificity

No data available
False positives can occur
    In infarcts
    In cysts

References

1. Berk, R. N., and Wholey, M. H. The application of splenic arteriography in the diagnosis of rupture of the spleen. *AJR* 104:662,
   1968.
2. Broderick, T. W. Contrast Material Reactions. In G. W. Friedland,
   R. Filly, and M. L. Goris (Eds.). *Uroradiology.* New York: Churchill
   Livingstone, 1983.
3. Federle, M. P., Goldberg, H. I., Kaiser, J. A., et al. Evaluation of
   abdominal trauma by computed tomography. *Radiology* 138:637,
   1981.
4. Froelich, J. W., Simeone, J. F., McKusick, K. A., et al. Radionuclide
   imaging and ultrasound in liver/spleen trauma: A prospective comparison. *Radiology* 145:457, 1982.
5. Gilday, D. L., and Alderson, P. O. Scintigraphic evaluation of liver
   and spleen injury. *Semin. Nucl. Med.* 4:357, 1974.
6. Hessel, S. J. Complications of Angiography and Other Catheter
   Procedures. In H. L. Abrams (Ed.). *Abrams Angiography: Vascular
   and Interventional Radiology* (3rd ed.). Boston: Little, Brown, 1983.
7. Jeffrey, R. B., Laing, F. C., Federle, M. P., et al. Computed tomography of splenic trauma. *Radiology* 141:729, 1981.
8. Love, L., Greenfield, G. B., Braun, T. W., et al. Arteriography of
   splenic trauma. *Radiology* 91:96, 1968.
9. Lutzker, L. G. Radionuclide imaging of the injured spleen and liver.
   Semin. Nucl. Med. 13:184, 1983.

Genitourinary Disease

Hematuria

Harry Z. Mellins

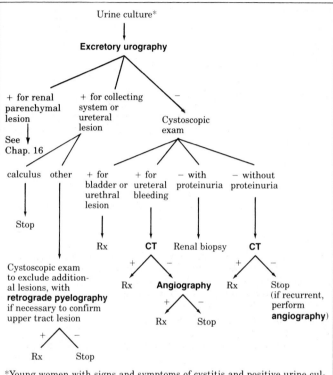

*Young women with signs and symptoms of cystitis and positive urine cultures should be treated without radiological examination. Successful treatment eliminates the need for further investigation

Typical Patient

Individual describing grossly bloody urine or whose urinalysis specimen reveals red blood cells

Typical Disorder(s)

Infections, calculi, obstruction, vascular lesions, and tumors involving the kidneys, ureters, bladder, and urethra

Comment

About 60% of cases are due to bleeding from the lower or mid-urinary tracts

Excretory Urography

Furnishes the broadest range of information of any urinary tract imaging examination

Drawbacks

Rare complications; occasional contrast reactions and/or secondary renal failure occur, with serious contrast reactions only 1 in 14,000 [2]

Peristalsis may prevent visualization of portions of the urinary tract, particularly the ureters; retrograde pyelography may be necessary to supplement excretory urography

If there is renal insufficiency, ultrasound will indicate renal size and will exclude hydronephrosis; retrograde pyelography may be necessary if detailed delineation of the upper tracts is required

Comments

Satisfactory renal function is required, although if higher contrast doses are used (which increase the risk of nephrotoxicity), some information can be produced with poor renal function

Sensitivity

Excretion urogram is abnormal in 67% of gross hematuria cases; in 40% of microscopic hematuria cases [5]

No precise data on sensitivity but relatively high for masses and stones (only a few cases of masses missed by excretion urography have been reported) [6]

False negatives can occur from
> Poor intestinal preparation
> Technically poor examination or an imprecise examination protocol

Specificity

No precise data available, but high

False positives can occur
> If normal variant (column of Bertin) is thought to be an abnormal mass

Retrograde Pyelography

Reveals the position and shape of the lumen of the upper urinary tracts when excretory urography is not desired (e.g., renal insufficiency, drug idiosyncrasy)

Permits taking urine samples from each ureter to be examined for blood or tumor cells

Permits brush biopsies to be taken

Drawbacks

Small risk of infection
Rare iatrogenic injuries (perforations) and sepsis

Comment

Requires preliminary cystoscopic examination

Sensitivity

For collecting system lesions: very high
For renal parenchymal lesions: much less sensitive than excretory urography
False negatives can occur
    If small parenchymal lesions do not impinge on pelvocalyceal system or alter renal outlines
    If there are small pelvic lesions and overdistention with too dense contrast material

Specificity

For collecting system lesions: very high
For renal parenchymal lesions: much less specific than excretory urography

Computed Tomography (CT)

See discussion in Chapter 10, p. 51

Renal Angiography

See discussion in Chapter 10, p. 51

Contribution of Magnetic Resonance Imaging [3, 4]

Distinguishes cyst from renal masses
May be useful in defining bladder pathology in general and bladder tumors in particular

References

1. Benson, G. S., and Brewer, E. D. Hematuria: Algorithms for diagnosis. II. Hematuria in the adult and hematuria secondary to trauma. *JAMA* 246:993, 1981.
2. Broderick, T. W. Contrast Material Reactions. In G. W. Friedland, R. Filly, and M. L. Goris (Eds.). *Uroradiology.* New York: Churchill Livingstone, 1983.
3. Bryan, P. J., Butler, H. E., LiPuma, J. P., et al. NMR scanning of the pelvis: Initial experience with a 0.3 T system. *AJR* 141:1111, 1983.

4. Choyke, P. L., Kressel, H. Y., Pollack, H. M., et al. Focal renal masses: Magnetic resonance imaging. *Radiology* 152:471, 1984.
5. Dana, A., Michel, J. R., Sterin, P., et al. Radiological investigations to establish etiology in patients with hematuria. A report on nearly 2,000 consecutive cases. *J. Radiol.* 61:585, 1980.
6. Kass, D. A., Hricak, H., and Davidson, A. J. Renal malignancies with normal excretory urograms. *AJR* 141:731, 1983.
7. Mellins, H. Z., McNeil, B. J., Abrams, H. L., et al. The selection of patients for excretory urography. *Radiology* 130:293, 1979.

14

Unexplained Renal Insufficiency/Failure

Peter M. Doubilet

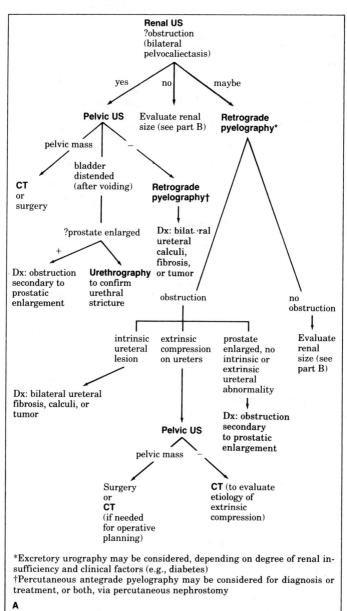

*Excretory urography may be considered, depending on degree of renal insufficiency and clinical factors (e.g., diabetes)
†Percutaneous antegrade pyelography may be considered for diagnosis or treatment, or both, via percutaneous nephrostomy

A

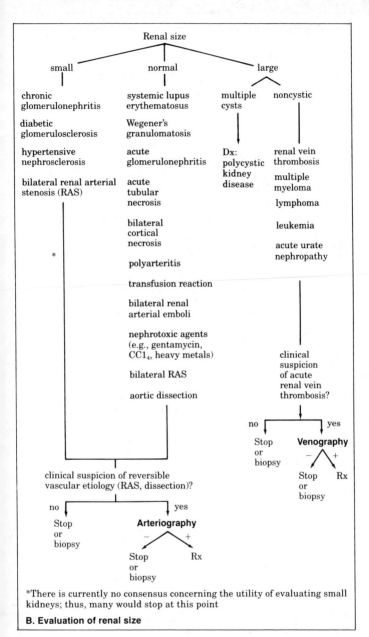

*There is currently no consensus concerning the utility of evaluating small kidneys; thus, many would stop at this point

B. Evaluation of renal size

Individual whose renal function tests indicate newly discovered renal insufficiency or failure (i.e., elevated BUN and creatinine and, frequently, decreased urine output) for uncertain reasons

Typical Disorder(s)

Postrenal obstruction: bilateral ureteral obstruction (e.g., pelvic mass, calculi, fibrosis)

Renal artery stenosis or emboli (bilateral)

Intrinsic renal diseases: polycystic kidney disease, acute glomerulonephritis, acute tubular necrosis, diabetic nephropathy

Comments

This algorithm does not address transplant renal insufficiency/failure

No imaging study may be needed when etiologies can be specified with confidence (e.g., patients with low cardiac output following myocardial infarction or those with active lupus)

No imaging study may be needed for women without pelvic masses because obstruction to urine outflow (the major reversible etiology to be excluded) is rare for such patients

Ultrasound (US)

Diagnoses obstruction and determines its etiology, if caused by a pelvic mass

Can be performed independent of renal function

Comments

A full bladder is required for the pelvic portion of the examination; catheterization may be required if the patient is anuric or severely oliguric

Image quality is better with thin patients, but hydronephrosis and pelvic mass generally can be diagnosed in spite of obesity.

Sensitivity

For obstruction: *98%* [1, 4]

False negatives can occur

    If dilated calyces are mistaken for cysts (poor technique)

    If obstruction is recent and acute, with minimal dilatation

Specificity

If mild hydronephrosis on ultrasound is interpreted as abnormal: *74–92%* [1, 4]

If mild hydronephrosis on ultrasound is interpreted as normal: *97%* [4]

False positives can occur if
> In the absence of obstruction there is a mild fullness of the collecting system sometimes related to the state of hydration
>
> Following pregnancy there is residual dilatation
>
> Full bladder leads to dilatation of renal pelvocalyceal system

Computed Tomography (CT)

Diagnoses location and presence of disease
Can detect unrelated abnormalities elsewhere

Drawbacks

Rare complications; occasional contrast reactions and/or secondary renal failure occur, with serious reactions only 1 in 14,000 [3]

Sensitivity

Yield in determining etiology of known hydronephrosis: *92%* [2]
False negatives can occur
> In the absence of gross mass, fibrosis, or tumor if infiltration of ureter goes undetected

Specificity

High (no precise data available)

Retrograde Pyelography

Provides definitive information concerning presence and location or absence of ureteral obstruction
May suggest the nature of the obstructing lesion

Drawbacks

Requires cystoscopic insertion and ureteral catheterization by a urologist
Requires general anesthesia and a 12-hour fast
Possible (rare) ureteral perforation, sepsis, contrast reactions, or temporary ureterovesical junction obstruction due to edema [5]

Sensitivity

For ureteral obstruction: approaching *100%*
False negatives can occur
> From poor technique

Specificity

For ureteral obstruction: approaching *100%*

False positives can occur
   From poor technique

Urethrography (Retrograde and Voiding Cystourethrography)

Definitive procedure for urethral pathology
Identifies presence and location of urethral stricture

Drawbacks

Uncomfortable
Infrequent sepsis or contrast extravasation [11]

Sensitivity

For urethral stricture: approaching *100%*
False negatives can occur
   From poor technique

Specificity

For urethral stricture: approaching *100%*
False positives can occur
   From poor technique

Arteriography/Venography

Required prior to surgical treatment of renal artery stenosis, aortic dissection, or acute renal vein thrombosis
Provides excellent detail of vascular anatomy
Arterial digital subtraction angiography may be used as an alternative because of smaller volume of contrast required

Drawbacks

Invasive, uncomfortable, requires hospitalization
Complications: Contrast reaction and/or secondary renal failure, rare; vascular injury and thrombosis, serious, about 1%; local hemorrhage or hematoma, nonfatal serious reactions, less than 2%; fatalities, .03% [6]. (Note: Vascular injury and thrombosis and local hematoma occur more frequently following arteriography than venography.)

Sensitivity

Approaching *100%*

Specificity

Approaching *100%*

Contribution of Magnetic Resonance Imaging [8]

Well demonstrates hydronephrosis
May distinguish vascular from nonvascular etiology
May play a role in differentiating acute tubular necrosis from other causes of renal insufficiency because of its capacity to define cortex and medulla

References

1. Arafa, N. M., Fathi, M. M., Safwat, M., et al. Accuracy of ultrasound in the diagnosis of nonfunctioning kidneys. *J. Urol.* 128:1165, 1982.
2. Bosniak, M. A., Megibow, A. J., Ambos, M. A., et al. Computed tomography of ureteral obstruction. *AJR* 138:1107, 1982.
3. Broderick, T. W. Contrast Material Reactions. In G. W. Friedland, R. Filly, and M. L. Goris (Eds.). *Uroradiology.* New York: Churchill Livingstone, 1983.
4. Ellenbogen, P. H., Scheible, F. W., Talner, L. B., et al. Sensitivity of gray scale ultrasound in detecting urinary tract obstruction. *AJR* 130:731, 1978.
5. Gross, D. Retrograde Urography and Retrograde Loopography. In G. W. Friedland, R. Filly, and M. L. Goris (Eds.). *Uroradiology.* New York: Churchill Livingstone, 1983.
6. Hessel, S. J. Complications of Angiography and Other Catheter Procedures. In H. L. Abrams (Ed.,). *Abrams Angiography: Vascular and Interventional Radiology* (3rd ed.). Boston: Little, Brown, 1983. Pp. 1041–1055.
7. Lee, J. K. T., Baron, R. L., Melson, G. L., et al. Can real-time ultrasonography replace static B-scanning in the diagnosis of renal obstruction? *Radiology* 139:161, 1981.
8. Leung, A. W. L., Bydder, G. M., Steiner, R. E., et al. Magnetic resonance imaging of the kidneys. *AJR* 143:1215, 1984.
9. Libertino, J. A., Zinman, L., Breslin, D. J., et al. Renal artery revascularization: Restoration of renal function. *JAMA* 244:1340, 1980.
10. McAfee, J. G., Thomas, F. D., Grossman, Z., et al. Diagnosis of angiotensinogenic hypertension: The complementary roles of renal scintigraphy and the saralasin infusion test. *J. Nucl. Med.* 18:669, 1977.
11. Mellins, H. Z. Radiology of the Urinary Tract: Urography and Cystourethrography. In J. H. Harrison, R. F. Gittes, A. D. Perlmutter, et al. (Eds.). *Campbell's Urology* (4th ed.). Philadelphia: Saunders, 1978.

15

Renovascular Hypertension

Stuart C. Geller

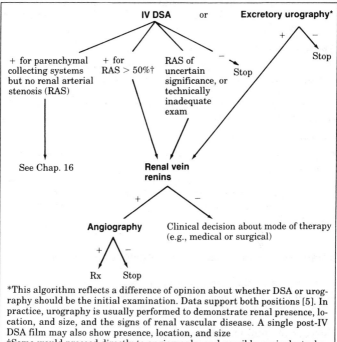

*This algorithm reflects a difference of opinion about whether DSA or urography should be the initial examination. Data support both positions [5]. In practice, urography is usually performed to demonstrate renal presence, location, and size, and the signs of renal vascular disease. A single post-IV DSA film may also show presence, location, and size

†Some would proceed directly to angiography and possible angioplasty, bypassing renal vein renins

Typical Patient

Individuals with systemic hypertension suspected of renovascular etiology, with systolic blood pressure more than 150 mm Hg and diastolic blood pressure more than 90 mm Hg. In addition one or more of the following conditions should also be present:

Poorly controlled hypertension on maximal medical therapy

Patient with severe hypertension and renal failure of obscure origin

Abdominal bruit

Recent recurrence of hypertension or increased control medication, following revascularization procedure

Suspected anastomotic stenosis following renal transplant

Elevated peripheral renins or other biochemical data indicating possible renovascular hypertension

Radiographic evidence (e.g., on intravenous or radionuclide urogram, ultrasound, CT scan) suggesting renovascular hypertension

Two or more medications required for control; disabling medication side effects and/or poor compliance; desire of patient and referring physician for definitive therapy if feasible

Typical Disorder(s)

Renal artery stenosis (most common etiologies: atherosclerotic disease, renal artery dysplasia, or postsurgical, i.e., anastomotic)

Functioning tumors (e.g., pheochromocytoma, renin secreting)

Essential hypertension

Comment

Renovascular hypertension may be secondary to causes other than renal artery stenosis, including parenchymal lesions such as cysts, tumors, scars, collecting system abnormalities, or arteriovenous malformations; these may be detected by use of this algorithm but are not the primary disorder being evaluated

Intravenous Digital Subtraction Angiography (IV DSA)

Exactly locates the lesion anatomically

In conjunction with poststudy abdominal radiography or distal nephropyelography can detect parenchymal and collecting system lesions

Surveys remaining abdominal vasculature

Less invasive than conventional aortography and can easily be used for outpatients

Drawbacks

Compared to conventional aortography:

Patient motion, bowel gas, or vascular overlap can significantly affect results

More contrast is necessary to obtain poorer quality information

Not as readily available and more operator-dependent

Not as reliable in diagnosing smaller vessel or branch stenoses

About 6–7% of the time examinations will be technically inadequate [5, 7]

Rare complications; occasional contrast reactions and/or secondary renal failure may occur, with serious reactions only 1 in 14,000 [2]

Comments

Patients should be able to withstand moderate amounts of iodinated intravenous contrast, have a normal cardiac output, have venous access, be free of excess bowel gas, be thin, and have had a clear liquid diet or NPO for 8–12 hours prior to the examination

IV DSA has been used in some centers to replace intravenous urography for diagnosing renovascular disease or for predicting therapeutic results; in fact, the contrast load of IV DSA is commonly used as a means of obtaining a urogram

Sensitivity

For detection of renal artery stenosis in those with a technically adequate examination: greater than 88% [5]

False negatives can occur

Because lower spatial resolution (compared to conventional aortography) prevents visualization of branch stenoses and small vessel lesions

If overlapping vessels obscure lesions

If other visceral branches are confused with renal arteries or a small field of view does not include an accessory renal artery

Specificity

For evaluating patients suspected of renal artery stenosis among those with technically adequate examinations: 90% [5]

False positives can occur from

Patient movement or bowel motion

Low spatial resolution

Quantum noise

A Mach effect from overlapping vessels

Excretory Urography

Demonstrates presence or absence of both kidneys

Demonstrates position and the relative sizes of both kidneys

Well-established criteria for diagnosis exist

May reflect physiological stigmata of renovascular hypertension, with hyperconcentration and delayed washout on involved side

Demonstrates nonvascular pathology, such as polycystic disease, tumor, hydronephrosis, that may be associated with hypertension

Drawbacks

Because of the known incidence of false negatives, urography—when negative—will sometimes be followed by digital subtraction angiography (DSA) if clinical suspicion is high. Alternatively, DSA may be used as the primary examination, as noted in the algorithm

Additional examination; sometimes considered unnecessary in some institutions

Comments

Excretory urography is an important diagnostic method for demonstrating parenchymal disease; the urogram sometimes reflects vascular disease without clarifying the precise condition of renal arteries and branches

Sensitivity

For detection of renal artery stenosis: 75% [5]
False negatives can occur
When the characteristic stigmata of renovascular hypertension such as delayed appearance time, hyperconcentration, and decreased size are not demonstrated (e.g., when disease is bilateral)
When rapid sequence filming is not performed

Specificity

For evaluating patients suspected of renal artery stenosis: 86% [1, 4]

Selective Renal Vein Renin Sampling

Determines a lesion's significance
Confirms successful surgical or angioplasty outcome (positive examination result predicts a successful therapy)
Can be performed simultaneously with other examination (IV DSA or aortography)

Drawbacks

High false negative ratio
Significant delay (days to weeks) between examination and results
Wide variation in assay techniques and interpretation of results

Comment

Optimally performed on those whose angiotensin-renin system has been stimulated (e.g., low sodium diets, 12 hours bed rest prior to examination, furosemide); who are not on medication that interferes with the renin; who have venous access (femoral preferable to supradiaphragmatic)

Sensitivity

To detect renovascular hypertension using ipsilateral-contralateral ratio of greater than or equal to 1.5: more than 90% [9]
To detect "curable" renovascular hypertension: quite variable, from 60% [9] to 90% [3]
False negatives can occur from
Bilateral renal artery stenosis
Branch renal artery stenosis
Inadequate prestudy stimulation of renin
Sampling site error

Too high blood pressure
Certain drugs (e.g., beta blockers, clonidine, possibly meth-
yldopa)

Specificity

Low: For evaluating patients suspected of renovascular disease,
only *60%* of patients subsequently shown to have essential
hypertension will have ipsilateral-contralateral ratios of less
than 1.5 [3]
False positives can occur
From parenchymal or collecting system abnormalities without renal artery stenosis

Aortography with Selective Renal Arteriography

Highly specific, serving as gold standard for diagnosing renal
artery stenosis
Allows further classification of stenosis etiology (i.e., fibromuscular disease vs. atherosclerosis)
Detects other renal parenchymal pathology, surveying vascular
disease elsewhere
Provides a road map for planning appropriate surgical revascularization procedure
Compared to IV DSA, uses less contrast to discover more information and has larger field of view plus biplane capability
Can perform diagnosis and therapy in same sitting (i.e., angioplasty)

Drawbacks

Complications: contrast reaction and/or secondary renal failure,
rare; vascular injury and thrombosis, serious, about 1%; local
hemorrhage or hematoma, nonfatal serious reactions, less
than 2%; fatalities, .03% [6]
Requires hospitalization for monitoring (for 8–12 hours); is
somewhat uncomfortable, usually needing analgesics; patient
must be able to tolerate moderate amounts of iodinated contrast

Comment

Requires intravenous line placement and arterial access (usually femoral)

Sensitivity

For detection of renal artery stenosis: *99%*
False negatives can occur
If accessory branches are missed
If a stenosis is concealed by overlapping branches

Specificity

For showing normal renal arteries: *99%*
False positives can occur
    With arterial spasm secondary to catheter placement

Contribution of Magnetic Resonance Imaging [8]

May demonstrate renal artery stenosis without contrast agent

References

1. Bookstein, J. J., Abrams, H. L., Buenger, R. E., et al. Radiologic aspects of renovascular hypertension. Part 2. The role of urography in unilateral renovascular disease. *JAMA* 220:1225, 1972.
2. Broderick, T. W. Contrast Material Reactions. In G. W. Friedland, R. Filly, and M. L. Goris (Eds.). *Uroradiology.* New York: Churchill Livingstone, 1983.
3. Buda, J. A., Baer, L., Parra-Carrillo, J. Z., et al. Predictability of surgical response in renovascular hypertension. *Arch. Surg.* 111:1243, 1976.
4. Erikson, U., Hemmingsson, A., Ljungström, A. et al. On the use of renal angiography and intravenous urography in the investigation of renovascular hypertension. *Acta Med. Scand.* 198:39, 1975.
5. Havey, R. J., Krumlovsky, F., delGreco, F., et al. Screening for renovascular hypertension. Is the renal DSA the preferred non-invasive test? *JAMA* 254:388, 1985.
6. Hessel, S. J. Complications of Angiography and Other Catheter Procedures. In H. L. Abrams (Ed.). *Abrams Angiography: Vascular and Interventional Radiology* (3rd ed.). Boston: Little, Brown, 1983. Pp. 1041–1055.
7. Hillman, B. J., Ovitt, T. W., Capp, M. P., et al. Renal digital subtraction angiography: 100 cases. *Radiology* 145:643, 1982.
8. Leung, A. W. L., Bydder, G. M., Steiner, R. E., et al. Magnetic resonance imaging of the kidneys. *AJR* 143:1215, 1984.
9. Maxwell, M. H., Marks, L. S., Lupu, A. N., et al. Predictive value of renin determinations in renal artery stenosis. *JAMA* 238: 2617, 1977.
10. McNeil, B. J. Varady, P. D. Burrows, B. A., et al. Measures of clinical efficacy. Cost-effectiveness calculations in the diagnosis and treatment of renovascular disease. *N. Engl. J. Med.* 293:216, 1975.
11. Smith, C. W., Winfield, A. C., Price, R. R., et al. Evaluation of digital venous angiography for the diagnosis of renovascular hypertension. *Radiology* 144:51, 1982.
12. Thornbury, J. R., Stanley, J. C., and Fryback, D. G. Hypertensive urogram: A nondiscriminatory test for renovascular hypertension. *AJR* 138:43, 1982.

Upper Urinary Tract Injury Following Trauma

Dana A. Twible

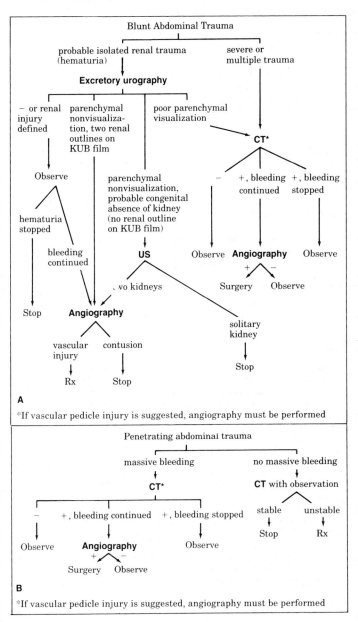

A

*If vascular pedicle injury is suggested, angiography must be performed

B

*If vascular pedicle injury is suggested, angiography must be performed

Typical Patient

Individual who has been in an accident (e.g., car crash, assault) that caused physical injury to the abdomen and who is brought to the emergency room

Typical Disorder(s)

Renal injury from blunt abdominal trauma and penetrating abdominal trauma [13]
    Major: parenchymal laceration, fracture, pelvocalyceal and ureteral injury
    Minor: contusions, forniceal rupture
    Critical: shattered kidney, vascular injury

Comment

Appropriate treatment depends on the extent of parenchymal, urinary tract, and vascular damage plus the hemodynamic status of the patient [7, 14]

Excretory Urography

Evaluates both anatomical integrity and physiological functioning of kidneys
Good screening examination to rule out serious renal injury

Drawbacks

Rare complications; occasional contrast reactions and/or secondary renal failure occur, with serious reactions only 1 in 14,000 [2]

Comments

If examination results are normal or if minor injury is demonstrated, no further work-up is necessary [7, 13]
Radionuclide renal scans may be substituted for excretory urography [4], especially for patients with contrast allergies

Sensitivity

About *90%* [4, 12]
False negatives can occur
    If minor injuries (e.g., contusion) or arteriovenous fistulas and traumatic renal artery aneurysms are not detected

Specificity

High when equivocal findings are excluded; otherwise, moderate [4, 12]
False positives can occur
    If there are causes other than vascular trauma (e.g., congenital absence, chronic obstruction, chronic infection, or contusion)

Computed Tomography (CT)

Provides good morphologic evidence of kidney injury extent, particularly perirenal and intrarenal hematomas and extravasation

Provides information about vascular perfusion of the kidney [9]

Evaluates multiple organ systems for injury

Drawbacks

Patient motion can seriously degrade image quality

Rare complications; occasionally contrast reactions and/or secondary renal failure occur, but serious reactions only 1 in 14,000 [2]

Sensitivity

More sensitive than excretion urography—about *20%* of patients with trauma will have additional or more specific findings (e.g., extravasation) seen on CT [11]

Specificity

High, and more specific than excretory urography

Ultrasound (US)

Provides anatomical, not functional, information about kidney: is limited, in this setting, to situations in which congenital absence of a kidney is suspected on the basis of nonvisualization on excretory urogram

Sensitivity

For diagnosis of congenital absence of kidney: approaching *100%*

Specificity

Very high

False positives can occur

   In atrophic pyelonephritis or pelvic kidney

Angiography

Provides the most accurate assessment of renal vasculature; is gold standard for comparison [10]

For acute renal trauma, can evaluate the cause of parenchymal nonvisualization on excretory urography or locate the cause of uncontrolled hemorrhage [10]

For chronic renal trauma, can diagnose arteriovenous fistulas or pseudoaneurysms [7]

Drawbacks

Complications: contrast reaction and/or secondary renal failure, rare; vascular injury and thrombosis, serious, about 1%; local hemorrhage or hematoma, nonfatal serious reactions, less than 2%; fatalities, .03% [8]

Sensitivity

Very high, approaching *100%* [4]
False negatives can occur
    If a vascular spasm delays recognizing a transection of a renal artery

Specificity

Very high, approaching *100%*
False positives can occur
    If a vascular spasm is mistaken for transection or occlusion of a normal renal artery

References

1. Ansell, G., Tweedie, M. C. K., West, C. R., et al. The current status of reactions to intravenous contrast media. *Invest. Radiol.* 15(Suppl.):S32, 1980.
2. Broderick, T. W. Contrast Material Reactions. In G. W. Friedland, R. Filly, and M. L. Goris (Eds.). *Uroradiology.* New York: Churchill Livingstone, 1983.
3. Byrd, L., and Sherman, R. L. Radiocontrast-induced acute renal failure: A clinical and pathophysiologic review. *Medicine* 58:270, 1979.
4. Chopp, R. T., Hekmat-Ravan, H., and Mendez, R. Technetium-99m glucoheptonate renal scan in diagnosis of acute renal injury. *Urology* 15:201, 1980.
5. Diaz-Buxo, J. A., Wagoner, R. D., Hattery, R. R., et al. Acute renal failure after excretory urography in diabetic patients. *Ann. Intern. Med.* 83:155, 1975.
6. Griffen, W. O., Belin, R. P., Ernst, C. B., et al. Intravenous pyelography in abdominal trauma. *J. Trauma* 18:387, 1978.
7. Guerriero, W. G. Trauma to the kidneys, ureters, bladder, and urethra. *Surg. Clin. North Am.* 62:1047, 1982.
8. Hessel, S. J. Complications of Angiography and Other Catheter Procedures. In H. L. Abrams (Ed.). *Abrams Angiography: Vascular and Interventional Radiology* (3rd ed.). Boston: Little, Brown, Pp. 1041–1055, 1983.
9. Lang, E. K. Assessment of renal trauma by dynamic computed tomography. *Radiographics* 3:566, 1983.
10. Lang, E. K., Trichel, B. E., Turner, R. W., et al. Arteriographic assessment of injury resulting from renal trauma. An analysis of 74 patients. *J. Urol.* 106:1, 1971.
11. McAninch, J. W., and Federle, M. P. Evaluation of renal injuries with computerized tomography. *J. Urol.* 128:456, 1982.
12. Morrow, J. W., and Mendez, R. Renal trauma. *J. Urol.* 104:649, 1970.

13. Moss, D. I., and Freeman, R. Renal angiography and the management of severe closed renal trauma. *Aust. N. Z. Surg.* 47:462, 1977.
14. Sargent, J. C., and Marquardt, C. R. Renal injuries. *J. Urol.* 63:1, 1950.
15. Segalowsky, A. I., McConnell, J. D., and Peters, P. C. Renal trauma requiring surgery: An analysis of 185 cases. *J. Trauma* 23:128, 1983.

Lower Urinary Tract Injury Following Trauma

Dana A. Twible and Peter M. Doubilet

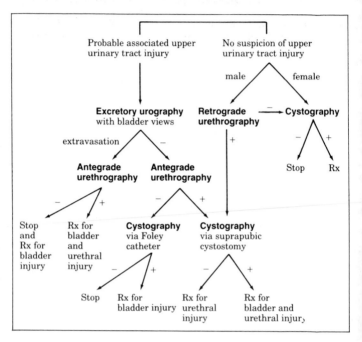

Typical Patient

Individual who has had blunt abdominal or pelvic trauma (e.g., accident, falling object) and is suspected of having a lower urinary tract injury

Typical Disorder(s)

Bladder rupture (intra- or extraperitoneal)
Posterior urethral rupture

Comments

Rupture of the posterior urethra is associated with bladder rupture about 16% of the time in males [3]; posterior urethral rupture is rare in females [5]

About 95% of patients with extraperitoneal bladder ruptures and 68% of those with intraperitoneal bladder ruptures have pelvic fractures [3]

Excretory Urography

Evaluates the upper urinary tract (kidneys and ureters) when associated injury to this area is suspected

May also allow examination of lower urinary tract if there is sufficient bladder distention

Drawbacks

Only about 15% of bladder injuries will be detected because of the failure to achieve adequate distention [5]

Sensitivity

87% for renal injury [1]

100% for ureteral injuries (when combined with retrograde pyelogram, if necessary)

Specificity

No precise data available, but generally high

Urethrography (Antegrade or Retrograde)

Retrograde urethrography must precede urethral catheterization (for cystography) in a patient with suspected urethral rupture

Antegrade urethrography can be performed following excretory urography, if the latter examination was obtained for suspected upper tract injury

Sensitivity

Approaching *100%* [1]

False negatives for posterior urethral rupture can occur with retrograde urethrography if the external sphincter remains closed [2]

Specificity

Approaching *100%*

Cystography

Mandatory for suspected bladder rupture (unless diagnosis of bladder rupture has been made by prior excretory urogram)

Drawbacks

Possible complications: cystitis, peritonitis, and infection of pelvic hematoma

Comments

Bladder is filled with contrast via urethral catheter, unless there is urethral rupture; if so, contrast is instilled via suprapubic needle

Sensitivity

For intraperitoneal rupture: approaching *100%* [1]
For extraperitoneal rupture: about *90%* [1]
False negatives can occur
> If a blood clot plugs the rupture
> If inadequate volumes of contrast are used

Specificity

For both intra- and extraperitoneal rupture: approaching *100%* [1]

References

1. Cass, A. S. Immediate radiological evaluation and early surgical management of genitourinary injuries from external trauma. *J. Urol.* 122:772, 1979.
2. Colapinto, V. Trauma to the pelvis: Urethral injury. *Clin. Orthopaed. Rel. Res.* 151:46, 1980.
3. Hayes, E. E., Sandler, C. M., and Corriere, J. N., Jr. Management of the ruptured bladder secondary to blunt abdominal trauma. *J. Urol.* 129: 946, 1983.
4. McLaughlin, A. P., III, and Pfister, R. C. Double catheter technique for evaluation of urethral injury and differentiating urethral from bladder rupture. *Radiology* 110:716, 1974.
5. Sandler, C. M., Phillips, J. M., Harris, J. D., et al. Radiology of the bladder and urethra in blunt pelvic trauma. *Radiol. Clin. North Am.* 19:195, 1981.

Differential Diagnosis of Scrotal Mass

William D. Kaplan and Jerome P. Richie

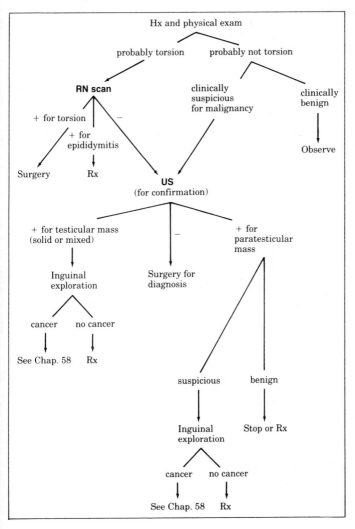

Typical Patient

Individual with either painful or painless scrotal mass

Typical Disorder(s)

Benign: testicular torsion, missed torsion, epididymitis, varico-
cele, hydrocele, orchitis (abscess)
Malignant: carcinoma, seminoma

Radionuclide (RN) Scan

Differentiates between torsion and acute epididymitis

Drawbacks

Inadequate for evaluation and staging of scrotal malignancy

Comment

Findings for torsion depend on the degree and duration of symptoms

Sensitivity

For torsion: greater than *95%* [3–5]
For epididymitis: *98%* [7]
False negatives can occur
    With early torsion (less than 5–7 hours)
    From technically inadequate examination resulting from
    poor counts, poor positioning, or inadequate magnifica-
    tion of testes

Specificity

Difficult if not impossible to determine: few afflicted patients
have surgery for clarification; however, probably
    Nearly *100%* for defining normal testes
    Nearly *100%* in differentiating acute epididymitis from
    acute torsion [3]
    About *75%* in differentiating abscess from slowly resolving
    epididymitis [3]

Ultrasound (US)

Differentiates between intratesticular and paratesticular pathology
Differentiates between solid, cystic, or mixed masses

Drawbacks

Does not reliably distinguish between benign and malignant
testicular masses
Does not reliably distinguish between early epididymitis and
acute testicular torsion

Sensitivity

For intratesticular vs. paratesticular: *80–90%* [6–8]
For solid vs. cystic vs. mixed: *96%* [6]

Specificity

For differentiating normal from abnormal: very high [6]
False positives can occur
> If cysts, giant orchitis, or hemangioendotheliomas are incorrectly thought to be tumors [7]

References

1. Boyce, W. H., and Politano, V. A. Infections and Disease of the Scrotum and Its Contents. In M. F. Campbell and J. H. Harrison (Eds.). *Urology.* Philadelphia: Saunders, 1970. Pp. 585–640.
2. Holder, L. E., Melloul, M., and Chen, D. Current status of radionuclide scrotal imaging. *Semin. Nucl. Med.* 11:232, 1981.
3. Holder, L. E., Martire, J. R., Holmes, E. R., III, et al. Testicular radionuclide angiography and static imaging: Anatomy, scintigraphic interpretation and clinical indications. *Radiology* 125:739, 1977.
4. Kogan, S. J., Lutzker, L. G., Perez, L. A., et al. The value of the negative radionuclide scrotal scan in the management of the acutely inflamed scrotum in children. *J. Urol.* 122:223, 1979.
5. Mendel, J., and Treves, T. Personal communication.
6. Orr, D. P., and Skolnick, M. L. Sonographic examination of the abnormal scrotum. *Clin. Radiol.* 31:109, 1980.
7. Richie, J. P., Birnholz, J., and Garnick, M. B. Ultrasonography as a diagnostic adjunct for the evaluation of masses in the scrotum. *Surg. Gynecol. Obstet.* 154:695, 1982.
8. Sample, W. F., Gottesman, J. E., Skinner, D. G., et al. Gray scale ultrasound of the scrotum. *Radiology* 127:225, 1978.
9. Stage, K. H., Schoenvogel, R., and Lewis, S. Testicular scanning: Clinical experience with 72 patients. *J. Urol.* 125:334, 1981.

Acute Testicular Pain

Sabah S. Tumeh

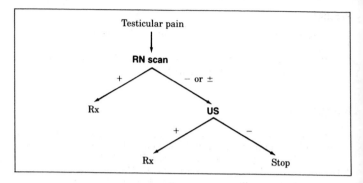

Typical Patient

Individual experiencing acute scrotal pain

Typical Disorder(s)

Torsion of testis
Torsion of testicular appendix
Epididymo-orchitis
Abscess

Radionuclide Scrotal Scan

Clarifies nature of problem rapidly (less than 15 minutes) to permit immediate surgical intervention should torsion be present

Using perfusion study followed by several static images allows torsion, epididymitis, and normal testis to be differentiated

Comments

Best for acute state

Sensitivity

For identifying acute torsion: *95%* [2–4]
False negatives can occur
> From a technically inadequate examination: poor counts, poor positioning, or insufficient magnification of testes

Specificity

For defining normal testes: approaching *100%*
For differentiating acute epididymitis from acute torsion: approaching *100%*

For differentiating abscess from slowly resolving epididymitis: about 75% [2]
False positives can occur
    If blood supply is compromised from other causes

Testicular Ultrasound (US)

Better for subacute (missed torsion) conditions, i.e., 1–10 days after symptomatology
In acute conditions (less than 6 hours of pain), findings are subtle

Sensitivity

For missed torsion: very high [4]
False negatives can occur
    If pain interferes with examination
    In the presence of reactive hydrocele

Specificity

For normal testes: very high if completely normal study is obtained in patients with symptoms for more than 6 hours
For distinguishing missed torsion from other diseases when characteristic features are present (disrupted parenchyma and globular epididymitis): very high [1]

References

1. Bird, K., Rosenfield, A. T., Taylor, K. J. W. Ultrasonography in testicular torsion. *Radiology* 147:527, 1983.
2. Holder, L. E., Martire, J. R., Holmes, E. R., III, et al. Testicular radionuclide angiography and static imaging: Anatomy, scintigraphic interpretation and clinical indications. *Radiology* 125:739, 1977.
3. Kogan, S. J., Lutzker, L. G., Perez, L. A., et al. The value of the negative radionuclide scrotal scan in the management of the acutely inflamed scrotum in children. *J. Urol.* 122:223, 1979.
4. Mendel, J., and Treves, T. Personal communication.

III

Chest Disease

Chest Pain, Probably Cardiac in Origin

David C. Levin

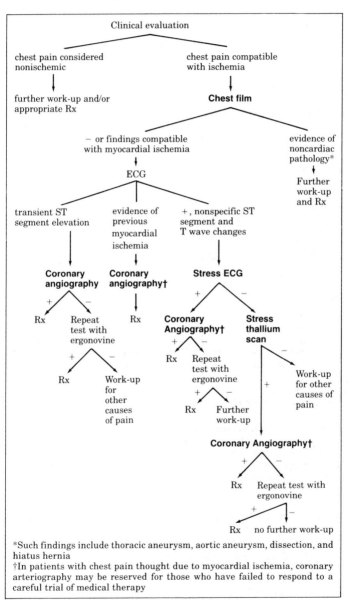

*Such findings include thoracic aneurysm, aortic aneurysm, dissection, and hiatus hernia

†In patients with chest pain thought due to myocardial ischemia, coronary arteriography may be reserved for those who have failed to respond to a careful trial of medical therapy

Typical Patient

Individual experiencing chest pain usually but not always related to exertion, which may radiate to the jaw or left arm,
and which may be associated with episodes of exertional dys-
pnea

Typical Disorder(s)

Obstructive coronary artery disease

Plain Chest Film

Assesses overall cardiac size, regional contour abnormalities,
and coronary artery calcification
Visualizes pulmonary vascular pattern, which helps assess cardiac function

Drawbacks

Not highly sensitive

Sensitivity

Very low
False negatives can occur
> If coronary artery disease does not produce the changes in
> size or contour of the heart of cardiac function that can
> be manifested on the film

Specificity

Relatively low
False positives can occur
> If any disease producing left ventricular enlargement (e.g.,
> hypertension, valvular heart disease, cardiomyopathy)
> mimics the findings of coronary artery disease

Coronary Arteriography

Definitely demonstrates number, site, severity of coronary artery lesions, and regional and global left ventricular function
(by left ventriculography)
Gold standard for detecting and defining extent of coronary artery disease during life

Drawbacks

Unless clearly greater than 50%, the physiological effect of stenosis may be uncertain
There is demonstrable interobserver variability
Frequently underestimates the severity of stenosis as compared
with pathological examinations
CASS study data indicate a death rate of 0.14%, myocardial infarction of 0.22%, stroke in 0.08%, arterial thrombosis in

0.24%, and arterial dissection in 0.13% (numbers refer to procedures performed by the Judkins technique) [4]

Requires a sophisticated catheterization laboratory, not readily available everywhere

Bandlike stenoses may be extremely hard to visualize [1, 5, 9]

Comments

Fluids only by mouth for 8 hours prior to examination

Sensitivity

Very high

False negatives can occur

If lesions are missed because of suboptimal cine equipment or improper projections

Specificity

Very high

False positives can occur

If a spasm mimics the presence of an organic stenosis (very rare)

Stress Electrocardiography (ECG)

Drawbacks

Drug effects, ventricular hypertrophy, intraventricular conduction, bundle branch block, or previous myocardial infarctions can frequently result in equivocal findings

Sensitivity

Depends on cut-off criterion (e.g., less than or equal to 1 mm ST segment depression, less than or equal to 2 mm depression, etc.) and extent of coronary artery disease: overall about *60%*

Specificity

Depends on cut-off criterion: overall about *83%*

Comment

The probability of a particular result on stress ECG depends on the extent of coronary artery disease (1, 2, 3 vessel disease or left main disease) and the millimeters of ST segment depression [13] (Table 20-1)

Thallium Studies

Noninvasively assesses regional myocardial perfusion: depicts relative rather than absolute perfusion

Is usually combined with stress ECG to determine extent to which perfusion abnormalities at exercise improve at rest—distinguishes ischemia from infarction

Table 20-1. Probability of Positive Stress ECG in Patients with Coronary Artery Disease

Stress Result (mm ST depression)	Extent of CAD				
	No CAD	1VD	2VD	3VD	LMD
≥ 1	13.1	59.6	73.6	83.8	93.3
≥ 2	0.8	22.3	34.6	54.9	75.6
≥ 3	0	8.2	24.2	37.1	60.0

Drawbacks

Exercise needed may rarely trigger an episode of severe myocardial ischemia, infarction, or congestive heart failure

Right ventricle is only faintly visualized in most patients at rest (although it can be seen during exercise images); hence, examination cannot diagnose ischemia of right ventricle

Diagnosing ischemic changes in a region of previous infarction is sometimes difficult

Comments

Exercise study takes 4 hours: first images immediately after exercise with repeat views 3 hours later

Exercise facilities are needed and patient must be able to exercise sufficiently to raise the coronary blood flow significantly

Sensitivity

About 20% more sensitive than stress ECG: *80–90%* [11, 12]; best for detecting disease of left main artery, left anterior descending artery, right anterior circumflex artery, and left circumflex artery, in that order

By using tomographic rather than planar imaging, sensitivity can be increased

False negatives can occur

    If well-developed collateral circulation obscures perfusion defects

    In patients on beta blockers

    If exercise images are not taken immediately after exercise (thallium may redistribute rapidly)

    In patients with single vessel disease

Specificity

About 10% more specific than stress ECG: greater than *90%* [12]

False positives can occur

    If there is attenuation of lateral wall by diaphragm

    In women because of breast attenuation

    In subcritical stenosis (less than 50%) with myocardial bridging

    In aortic stenosis

Contribution of Magnetic Resonance Imaging [6, 7, 8, 10]

May demonstrate ischemic or infarcted myocardium, ventricular and aortic aneurysm, atheromatous plaques in walls of large arteries

References

1. Arnett, E. N., Isner, J. M., Redwood, D. R., et al. Coronary artery narrowing in coronary heart disease: Comparison of cineangiographic and necropsy findings. *Ann. Intern. Med.* 91:350, 1979.
2. Bodenheimer, M. M., Banka, V. S., Fooshee, C., et al. Relationship between regional myocardial perfusion and the presence, severity and reversibility of asynergy in patients with coronary heart disease. *Circulation* 58:789, 1978.
3. Doubilet, P., McNeil, B. J., Weinstein, M. C. The decision concerning coronary angiography in patients with chest pain: A cost-effectiveness analysis. *Med. Decision Making* In press, 1985.
4. Davis, K., Kennedy, J. W., Kemp, H. G., et al. Complications of coronary arteriography from the collaborative study of coronary artery surgery (CASS). *Circulation* 59:1105, 1979.
5. Gronding, C. M., Dyrda, I., Pasternac, A., et al. Discrepancies between cineangiographic and postmortem findings in patients with coronary artery disease and recent myocardial revascularization. *Circulation* 49:703, 1974.
6. Herfkens, R. J., Higgins, C. B., Hricak, H., et al. Nuclear magnetic resonance imaging of the cardiovascular system: Normal and pathologic findings. *Radiology* 147:749, 1983.
7. Herfkens, R. J., Higgins, C. B., Hricak, H., et al. Nuclear magnetic resonance imaging of atherosclerotic disease. *Radiology* 148:161, 1983.
8. Higgins, C. B., Lanzer, P., Stark, D., et al. Imaging by nuclear magnetic resonance in patients with chronic ischemic heart disease. *Circulation* 69:523, 1984.
9. Hutchins, G. M., Bulkley, B. H., Ridolfi, R. L., et al. Correlation of coronary arteriograms and left ventriculograms with postmortem studies. *Circulation* 56:32, 1977.
10. Lieberman, J. M., Alfidi, R. J., Nelson, A. D., et al. Gated magnetic resonance imaging of the normal and diseased heart. *Radiology* 152:465, 1984.
11. Massie, B. M., Botvinick, E. H., and Brundage, B. H. Correlation of thallium-201 scintigrams with coronary anatomy: Factors affecting region by region sensitivity. *Am. J. Cardiol.* 44:616, 1979.
12. Okada, R. D., Boucher, C. A., Strauss, H. W., et al. Exercise radionuclide imaging approaches to coronary artery disease. *Am. J. Cardiol.* 46:1188, 1980.
13. Rigo, P., Beckar, L. C., Griffith, L. S. C., et al. Influence of coronary collateral vessels on the results of thallium-201 myocardial stress imaging. *Am. J. Cardiol.* 44:452, 1979.
14. Wainwright, R. J., Maisey, M. N., Edwards, A. C., et al. Functional significance of coronary collateral circulation during dynamic exercise evaluated by thallium-201 myocardial scintigraphy. *Br. Heart J.* 43:47, 1980.

Cardiomegaly

Michael F. Meyerovitz

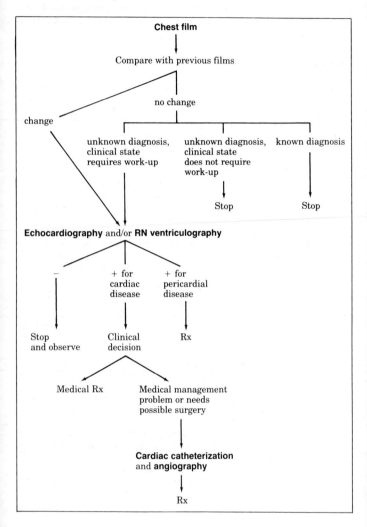

Typical Patient

Individual whose heart size has been determined to be large either on physical examination or on the chest radiograph

Typical Disorder(s)

Valvular, coronary (including aneurysm), cardiomyopathic, or congenital heart disease
Pericardial disease

Comment

When cardiomegaly is secondary to identifiable extracardiac causes (e.g., anemia, thyrotoxicosis), no further cardiac work-up is required

Plain Chest Film

Assesses overall cardiac size, regional contour abnormalities, coronary artery calcification, and pulmonary vascular pattern
Chamber enlargement allows assessment of the type of valvular disease
Pulmonary vascular pattern allows inferences of the presence of normal or increased pulmonary blood flow or pulmonary hypertension

Drawbacks

Cardiac chamber enlargement may be present without necessarily being reflected on conventional radiographs
Global view of the heart allows few precise statements about its internal anatomy
Distinctions of cardiomegaly etiology are not usually feasible (hypertension, valvular heart disease, ischemic disease, and cardiomyopathies occasionally produce similar radiographic patterns)

Comments

Chest films are most valuable in longitudinal studies of heart changes in a particular individual
The range of normal and abnormal heart size is great

Sensitivity

For pericardial effusions: 52% (using epicardial fat pad sign) [2]
For left ventricular aneurysm: 62% [8]
For acquired and congenital aortic valve stenosis or insufficiency: 93% (using bulging of lower third of left cardiac border) [11]
For mitral stenosis: 97% (using left atrial enlargement) [3]
For uncomplicated coronary disease: low

Specificity

For differentiating normal size heart from enlarged heart: high
False positives for cardiac disease can occur
    When heart is enlarged because of extracardiac conditions

Echocardiography

Assesses valvular motion and chamber size
Excellent means of identifying pericardial disease
Rapid and relatively accurate in experienced hands
Procedure of choice for asymmetric septal hypertrophy

Drawbacks

Adequate visualization of all structures is sometimes impossible

Comment

18% of left ventricular wall regions cannot be adequately visualized with echocardiography; in wall regions adequately visualized, wall motion characteristics are correctly identified 87% of the time, compared to biplane cine ventriculography [10]

Sensitivity

For asymmetric septal hypertrophy: approaching *100%*
For left ventricular hypertrophy: *93%* [15]
For critical aortic stenosis: *91%* [5]
For pericardial effusion: high [9]
For uncomplicated coronary artery disease: low
False negatives can occur
    From observer error
    With inadequate visualization of target area
    With tangential angulation of transducer through short axis of ventricular cavity, resulting in distortion of wall motion [9]

Specificity

For differentiating normal from hypertrophied ventricles: *95%* [15]
For differentiating normal from stenotic valves: *65%* [5]
For differentiating normal pericardial sacs from those with effusions: high [9]

Radionuclide (RN) Ventriculography

Evaluates absolute and relative ventricular volume, ejection fraction, regurgitant index, and wall motion
Provides quantitative data
Noninvasively quantifies degree of valvular insufficiency, particularly in patients without compromised left ventricular function (ejection fractions less than 35%)

Sensitivity

For measuring ejection fractions: high—correlation of 0.8–0.9 with results of cine angiography [1]
For left ventricular aneurysms: *95%* [7]

For detecting left-sided valvular regurgitation: for 1 + regurgitation, *85%;* for 2 + or more, *92%* [7]
False negatives can occur, rarely,
> For inferior or inferoposterior aneurysms (seen best with steep LAO or LPO views)

Specificity

For differentiating normal ventricle from one with aneurysm: *97%* [7]
For differentiating normal valves from regurgitative valves: *98%* [14]

Cardiac Catheterization and Angiography

Precisely depicts internal anatomy of heart
Defines location and presence of disease
Permits pressure measurements

Drawbacks

Serious potential complications [4]: mortality, 0.14%; myocardial infarction, 0.22%; stroke, 0.08%; arterial thrombosis, 0.24%; arterial dissection (using Judkins technique), 0.13%
Often difficult to determine accurately the physiological significance of an anatomical abnormality

Sensitivity

For all diseases of interest, very high by definition: gold standard
False negatives can occur
> From foreshortening and overlapping of vessels
> From superimposition of abnormally contracting regions of ventricular wall on left ventriculography

Specificity

Very high by definition: gold standard
False positives can occur with
> Coronary artery spasm
> Coronary artery anomalies
> Myocardial bridges

Contribution of Magnetic Resonance Imaging [6, 12, 13]

Can assess overall heart and individual chamber size and wall thickness
Useful in diagnosing congenital and acquired disease, intracavitary neoplasms, pericardial thickening and effusion

References

1. Ashburn, W. L., Schelbert, H. R., and Verba, J. W. Left ventricular ejection fraction. A review of several radionuclide angiographic approaches using the scintillation camera. *Prog. Cardiovasc. Dis.* 20:267, 1978.
2. Carsky, E. W., Mauceri, R. A., and Azimi, F. The epicardial fat pad sign: Analysis of frontal and lateral chest radiographs in patients with pericardial effusion. *Radiology* 137:303, 1980.
3. Chen, J. T. T., Behar, V. S., Morris, J. J., Jr., et al. Correlation of roentgen findings with hemodynamic data in pure mitral stenosis. *AJR* 102:280, 1968.
4. Davis, K., Kennedy, J. W., Kemp, H. G., Jr., et al. Complications of coronary arteriography from the collaborative study of coronary artery surgery (CASS). *Circulation* 59:1105, 1979.
5. DeMaria, A. N., Bommer, W., Joye, J., et al. Value and limitations of cross-sectional echocardiography of the aortic valve in the diagnosis and quantification of valvular aortic stenosis. *Circulation* 62:304, 1980.
6. Fletcher, B. D., Jacobstein, M. D., Nelson, A. D., et al. Gated magnetic resonance imaging of congenital cardiac malformations. *Radiology* 150;137, 1984.
7. Friedman, M. L., and Cantor, R. E. Reliability of gated heart scintigrams for detection of left-ventricular aneurysm: Concise communication. *J. Nucl. Med.* 20:720, 1979.
8. Gorlin, R., Klein, M. D., and Sullivan, J. M. Prospective correlative study of ventricular aneurysm. Mechanistic concept and clinical recognition. *Am. J. Med.* 42:512, 1967.
9. Horowitz, M. S., Schultz, C. S., Stinson, E. G., et al. Sensitivity and specificity of echocardiographic diagnosis of pericardial effusion. *Circulation* 50:239, 1974.
10. Kisslo, J. A., Robertson, D., Gilbert, B. W., et al. A comparison of real-time, two-dimensional echocardiography and cineangiography in detecting left ventricular asynergy. *Circulation* 55:134, 1977.
11. Klatte, E. C., Tampas, J. P., Campbell, J. A., et al. The roentgenographic manifestations of aortic stenosis and aortic valvular insufficiency. *AJR* 88:57, 1962.
12. Lieberman, J. M., Alfidi, R. J., Nelson, A. D., et al. Gated magnetic resonance imaging of the normal and diseased heart. *Radiology* 152:465, 1984.
13. McNamara, M. I., and Higgins, C. B. Cardiovascular applications of magnetic resonance imaging. *Magnetic Resonance Imaging* 2:167, 1984.
14. Nicod, P., Corbett, J. R., Firth, B. G., et al. Radionuclide techniques for valvular regurgitant index: Comparison in patients with normal and depressed ventricular function. *J. Nucl. Med.* 23:763, 1982.
15. Reichek, N., Devereux, R. B. Left ventricular hypertrophy: Relationship of anatomic, echocardiographic and electrocardiographic findings. *Circulation* 63:1391, 1981.

Abnormality of the Contour of the Cardiomediastinal Silhouette

Lawrence M. Boxt

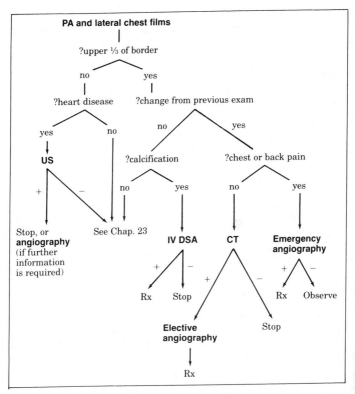

Typical Patient

Individual receiving posteroanterior and lateral chest examination, especially in emergencies

Typical Disorder(s)

Acute vascular emergencies
Leaking thoracic aortic aneurysm
Acute dissection of the thoracic aorta
For a stable patient: a problem of
Differentiating great vessels disease from mediastinal pathology
Differentiating cardiac from mediastinal disease

Posteroanterior (PA) and Lateral Chest Films

Provides familiar format (anatomical) of data presentation
Can be performed in any patient population

Sensitivity

For thoracic aortic dissection—with changes in aortic arch diameter between two examinations: about *82%* [13]

For acquired and congenital aortic valvular stenosis and insufficiency—with bulging of one-third of left cardiac border: *93%* [11]

For mitral stenosis—with left atrial enlargement with prominence of left heart border or posterior enlargement of atrium: *96%* [5]

For left ventricular aneurysm: *62%* [7]

False negatives can occur if
There are no previous films for comparison
Film is obtained in anteroposterior (AP) projection (i.e., portable or supine examination)

Specificity

Likely to be low—virtually any alteration of mediastinal anatomy will produce alteration on chest film

False positives can occur
With a thickened aorta or a congenital anomaly

Cardiac Ultrasound (US)

Useful for diagnosing valvular abnormalities
Demonstrates both severity and presence of lesion
Interactive, real time examination—highly observer dependent

Drawbacks

Recording and interpretation are sometimes difficult in patients with chronic obstructive pulmonary disease (COPD) or those with heavy calcium deposits on their aortic valve [6]

Sensitivity

For left ventricular hypertrophy: *93%* [12]
For aortic valvular stenosis: *91%* [6]
For left ventricular aneurysm: Small study only, but 4 out of 5 patients with LV aneurysm were documented by examination [4]

Specificity

For left ventricular hypertrophy: *95%* [12]
For aortic valvular stenosis: *65%* [6]
False positives can occur for aortic valvular stenosis
If left ventricular function is markedly impaired

Intravenous Digital Subtraction Angiography (IV DSA)

Confirms vascular abnormality or anomaly with less patient risk than does conventional aortography

Examination quality varies markedly with different equipment, contrast injection, and patient weight

Drawbacks

Patient may sustain potentially large contrast load

Rare complications; occasional contrast reactions and/or secondary renal failure may occur, with serious reactions only 1 in 14,000 [3]

Comments

Adequate left ventricular function is very helpful

Sensitivity

For thoracic aortic dissections: no data but probably low

For aneurysms: no data but probably very high

False negatives can occur for dissections

   If flap is out of imaging plane or is not thick enough to be resolved

Specificity

No data, but probably only moderate because of low spatial resolution

Computed Tomography (CT)

Used as screening procedure when aortic dissection is suspected

Contrast enhancement is essential

Dynamic studies with sequential slices are preferable

Drawbacks

Provides less information about aortic valve involvement, coronary arteries, or great vessels than does catheter angiography

Rare complications; occasional contrast reactions and/or secondary renal failure occur, but serious reactions only 1 in 14,000 [3]

Comments

CT as a screening procedure rarely suffices for patients being considered for surgery or dissection, and angiography generally follows; in stable patients, normal CT is considered adequate to exclude dissection

Sensitivity

For thoracic aortic dissections: limited data but probably about 85% [8]

For aneurysms: limited data but likely to be very high

False negatives can occur
  If no contrast is given

Specificity

Essentially no data on normal individuals studied with techniques more invasive than CT, but probably higher

Angiography

Identifies complete location of dissection
Provides "radiographic proof" of diagnosis or exclusion of disease

Drawbacks

Potentially hemodynamically destabilizing
Mortality: .03%; complications relating to examination, manipulation of aortic catheter, and/or contrast administration, including hematoma, arterial embolization, allergy-type reactions: 1–4% [10]

Comment

Adequate hydration and an 8- to 12-hour fast are helpful, if examination is elective

Sensitivity

For thoracic aortic dissections, using older published data: *80%* [13]; however, current practice with well-performed (biplane) examinations and with repeat injections of contrast, if necessary, is likely to be associated with sensitivity greater than *90%*
For thoracic aneurysms: very high
False negatives can occur
  If single plane rather than biplane imaging is performed

Specificity

Extremely high

Contribution of Magnetic Resonance Imaging [1, 2]

Delineates cardiac chambers and major blood vessels without use of contrast
Distinguishes vascular anomalies from mediastinal masses
Can assess the type and extent of aortic dissection, coarctation, aneurysms of the thoracic aorta

References

1. Amparo, E. G., Higgins, C. B., Farmer, D., et al. Gated MRI of cardiac and paracardiac masses: Initial experience. *AJR* 143:1151, 1984.
2. Amparo, E. G., Higgins, C. B., Hoddick, W., et al. Magnetic resonance imaging of aortic disease: Preliminary results. *AJR* 143:1203, 1984.
3. Broderick, T. W. Contrast Material Reactions. In G. W. Friedland, R. Filly, and M. L. Goris (Eds.). *Uroradiology.* New York: Churchill Livingstone, 1983.
4. Catherwood, E., Mintz, G. S., Kotler, M. N., et al. Two-dimensional echocardiographic recognition of left ventricular pseudoaneurysm. *Circulation* 62:294, 1980.
5. Chen, J. T. T., Behar, V. S., Morris, J. J., Jr., et al. Correlation of roentgen findings with hemodynamic data in pure mitral stenosis. *AJR* 102:280, 1968.
6. DeMaria, A. N., Bommer, W., Joye, J., et al. Value and limitations of cross-sectional echocardiography of the aortic valve in the diagnosis and quantification of valvular aortic stenosis. *Circulation* 62:304, 1980.
7. Gorlin, R., Klein, M. D., and Sullivan, J. M. Prospective correlative study of ventricular aneurysm. Mechanistic concept and clinical recognition. *Am. J. Med.* 42:512, 1967.
8. Heiberg, E., Wolverson, M., Sundaram, M., et al. CT findings in thoracic aortic dissection. *AJR* 136:136, 1981.
9. Hemley, S. D., Kanick, V., Kittredge, R. D., et al. Dissecting aneurysms of the thoracic aorta: Their angiographic demonstration. *AJR* 91:1263, 1964.
10. Hessel, S. J., Adams, D. F., and Abrams, H. L. Complications of angiography. *Radiology* 138:273, 1981.
11. Klatte, E. C., Tampas, J. P., Campbell, J. A., et al. The roentgenographic manifestations of aortic stenosis and aortic valvular insufficiency. *AJR* 88:57, 1962.
12. Reichek, N., and Devereux, R. B. Left ventricular hypertrophy: Relationship of anatomic, echocardiographic and electrocardiographic findings. *Circulation* 63:1391, 1981.
13. Wyman, S. M. Dissecting aneurysm of the thoracic aorta: Its roentgen recognition. *AJR* 78:247, 1957.

Radiographically Abnormal Mediastinum

Paul W. Spirn

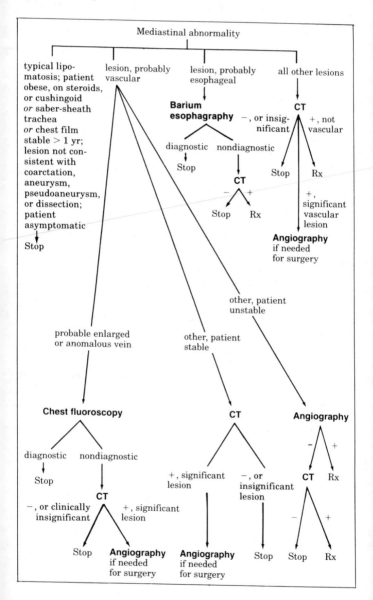

Typical Patient

Individual whose plain chest radiographs show an abnormality of the mediastinum: generalized or focal widening, an additional or distorted contour, or displacement or narrowing of the trachea

Typical Disorder(s)

Primary and metastatic malignancy, particularly bronchogenic and esophageal carcinoma, lymphoma, germ cell tumors, and thymoma

Aortic aneurysm, dissection, disruption, and coarctation

Congenital cysts, vascular anomalies

Benign variations that can mimic important abnormalities, such as intrathoracic goiter, vascular tortuosity, esophageal hiatus hernia, and asymmetric fat deposition

Barium Esophagography

Distinguishes intraluminal from extraluminal origin and determines extent of processes involving the esophagus

Drawbacks

Evaluation is limited to a relatively small sector of the mediastinum

Generally nonspecific in evaluating processes outside the esophagus

Sensitivity

For esophageal lesions: very high

False negatives can occur

> If mediastinal lesion does not impinge on esophagus

Specificity

For a normal esophagus: high

False positives can occur

> Because esophageal lumen may be distorted by normal vascular structures, and configuration varies with patient position and esophageal peristalsis

Computed Tomography (CT)

Localizes abnormality with regard to mediastinal compartments, often showing organ of origin and adjacent structure involvement

Crucial to planning diagnostic and therapeutic surgery and to staging

Broadly characterizes the physical constituency of an abnormality, often sufficiently to avoid invasive diagnostic or therapeutic procedures [3]

Simultaneously evaluates lungs, hila, pleural space, chest wall, and contiguous areas of the neck and upper abdomen for extension of mediastinal pathology or other pertinent abnormalities

Drawbacks

Rare complications; occasional contrast reactions and/or secondary renal failure occur, with serious reactions only 1 in 14,000 [4]

Comments

Requires patient to stay recumbent for 30–60 minutes and repeated short intervals of breath-holding
Scanning with contrast requires a tolerance to and access for intravenous contrast agents

Sensitivity

For detecting malignancy or neoplasm requiring surgery for diagnosis or treatment: *82%* [3]
For diagnosing vascular lesions: *92%* [3]
For diagnosing other nonvascular lesions: high
False negatives can occur
> Due to technical limitations of early-stage equipment
> If intravenous contrast is not administered correctly, when indicated [7]

Specificity

For ascertaining absence of malignancy (benign, normal, or vascular structure): *81%* [3]
False positives can occur
> Due to technical limitations of early-stage equipment
> Because reactive adenopathy, unless calcified, is indistinguishable from malignant adenopathy
> If intravenous contrast is not administered correctly, when indicated

Chest Fluoroscopy

Interactive examination permits precise localization of lesions
Distinguishes some vascular from nonvascular lesions
Patient maneuvers (e.g., Valsalva) must be performed under direct vision of radiologist

Drawbacks

Restricted to a small range of mediastinal venous abnormalities

Comments

Requires breath-holding maneuvers

Sensitivity and Specificity

For distinguishing some mediastinal venous abnormalities from other lesions: moderately high
False negatives and *false positives* can occur
    With an inexperienced operator

Thoracic Arteriography

Definitive study for exclusion and precise anatomical identification of all intrathoracic arterial abnormalities [1, 9]
Simultaneously evaluates associated cardiovascular lesions

Drawbacks

Complications: Contrast reaction and/or secondary renal failure, rare; serious vascular injury and thrombosis, about 1%; local hemorrhage or hematoma, nonfatal serious reactions, less than 2%; fatalities, .03% [8]

Comments

Requires catheter access to the thoracic aorta
Patient must have tolerance for intravascular contrast agent and no uncorrectable coagulopathy

Sensitivity

For aneurysm and aortic dissection: greater than *90%*
False negatives can occur
    Occasionally when aneurysm or dissection contains thrombus

Specificity

For showing normal vascular structures: high
False positives can occur
    In suspected dissection, when thrombosed false channel is mimicked by atherosclerotic intimal plaque, mural thrombus, or mediastinal fat

Contributions of Magnetic Resonance Imaging [5, 12]

Delineates mediastinal vascular abnormalities
Also defines cystic and solid mediastinal tumors
Its capacity for tissue characterization of benign versus malignant tumors is as yet undefined

References

1. Abrams, H. L., and Jönsson, G. Coarctation of the Aorta. In H. L. Abrams (Ed.). *Abrams Angiography: Vascular and Interventional Radiology* (3rd ed.). Boston: Little, Brown, 1983. Pp. 383–466.

2. Baron, R. L., Gutierrez, F. R., Sagel, S. S., et al. CT of anomalies of the mediastinal vessels. *AJR* 137:571, 1981.
3. Baron, R. L., Levitt, R. G., Sagel, S. S., et al. Computed tomography in the evaluation of mediastinal widening. *Radiology* 138:107, 1981.
4. Broderick, T. W. Contrast Material Reactions. In G. W. Friedland, R. Filly, and M. L. Goris (Eds.). *Uroradiology*. New York: Churchill Livingstone, 1983.
5. Gamsu, G., Stark, D. D., Webb, R., et al. Magnetic resonance imaging of benign mediastinal masses. *Radiology* 151:709, 1984.
6. Greene, R., and Lechner, G. L. "Saber-sheath" trachea: A clinical and functional study of marked coronal narrowing of the intrathoracic trachea. *Radiology* 115:265, 1975.
7. Godwin, J. D., Turley, K., Herfkens, R. J., et al. Computed tomography for follow-up of chronic aortic dissections. *Radiology* 139:655, 1981.
8. Hessel, S. J. Complications of Angiography and Other Catheter Procedures. In H. L. Abrams (Ed.). *Abrams Angiography: Vascular and Interventional Radiology* (3rd ed.). Boston: Little, Brown, 1983. Pp. 1041–1055.
9. Hynes, D. M., and Grainger, R. G. The angiographic demonstration of coarctation of aorta and similar anomalies. *Clin. Radiol.* 19:438, 1968.
10. Lee, W. J., and Fattal, G. Mediastinal lipomatosis in simple obesity. *Chest* 70:308, 1976.
11. Price, J. E., Jr., and Rigler, L. G. Widening of the mediastinum resulting from fat accumulation. *Radiology* 96:497, 1970.
12. Webb, W. R., Jensen, B. G., Gamsu, G., et al. Coronal magnetic resonance imaging of the chest: Normal and abnormal. *Radiology* 153:729, 1984.

Hilar Enlargement

Paul W. Spirn

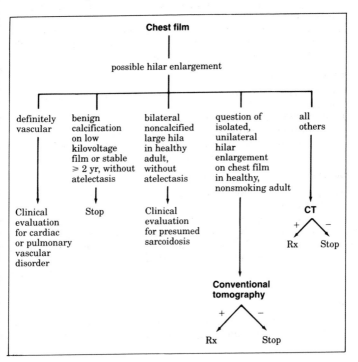

Chest film

|
possible hilar enlargement
|

definitely vascular → Clinical evaluation for cardiac or pulmonary vascular disorder

benign calcification on low kilovoltage film or stable ≥ 2 yr, without atelectasis → Stop

bilateral noncalcified large hila in healthy adult, without atelectasis → Clinical evaluation for presumed sarcoidosis

question of isolated, unilateral hilar enlargement on chest film in healthy, nonsmoking adult → **Conventional tomography** + Rx − Stop

all others → **CT** + Rx − Stop

Typical Patient

Individual whose chest radiograph suggests hilar enlargement
Individual with malignancy, known for hilar metastases, whose management would be influenced by the presence of adenopathy in hila that are normal or equivocal on chest radiographs

Typical Disorder(s)

Malignant: bronchogenic carcinoma, lymphoma, bronchial carcinoid, extrathoracic primary tumor metastasizing to chest
Nonmalignant: pulmonary arterial or venous dilation or tortuosity, cysts, granulomatous adenopathy including sarcoidosis, benign tumors

Plain Chest Film

Essential first step in hilar workup, ideally to compare with prior films

Comments

Noncalcified, bilateral hilar adenopathy as an isolated radiographic abnormality in an otherwise normal adult, with no history of prior malignancy, is presumed due to sarcoidosis [11]

Low kilovoltage radiographs can sometimes document the large quantity of nodal calcification needed to satisfy the radiographic criteria of benign granulomatous adenopathy

Sensitivity

For detecting hilar adenopathy in patients with lung cancer: average 57% [4, 8]

False negatives can occur because

Adjacent vascular structures are complex

Endobronchial lesions and early malignant adenopathy may not enlarge hilar outlines

Specificity

For indicating normal hila in patients with lung cancer: average 76% [4, 8]

False positives can occur

Because reactive and malignant adenopathy are often radiographically indistinguishable unless the former shows a benign pattern of calcification

Because vascular abnormalities, particularly when asymmetric, can simulate adenopathy

Comment

These sensitivity and specificity results can probably be exceeded if earlier radiographs are available for comparison

Computed Tomography (CT)

Capable of distinguishing vascular from other causes of hilar enlargement

Assesses lungs and mediastinum simultaneously

Helps direct a mediastinal or hilar biopsy procedure based on precise localization of enlarged lymph nodes

Obviates the need for mediastinal exploration before thoracotomy in patients with normal mediastinal CT who have known or suspected lung cancer [3]

Drawbacks

Rare complications; occasional contrast reactions and/or secondary renal failure occur, with serious reactions only 1 in 14,000 [2]

Adequate CT evaluation of the hilum requires third- or fourth-generation equipment with scanning times less than 10 seconds and collimation of 10 mm or less, and often requires the selective use of intravenous contrast agents

Requires skillful interpretation of a region of considerable anatomical complexity

Comments

In experienced hands, conventional and computed tomography are probably equally accurate for evaluation of the hila; the advantage of CT in clinical practice is its greater accuracy in mediastinal evaluation where there is frequently associated pathology that is more significant in terms of management and more accessible to biopsy than occurs in the hilar lesions

Sensitivity

For detecting malignant hilar adenopathy: average *81%* [4, 8]

For detecting malignant mediastinal adenopathy: average *94%* [5, 6, 8]

False negatives can occur

> If high resolution technique is not used or if administration of intravenous contrast agent is not properly timed

> Because early malignant adenopathy may not enlarge lymph nodes

Specificity

For indicating normal hila in patients with possible malignancy: average *88%* [4, 8]

For indicating normal mediastinum in patients with lung cancer: average *73%* [5, 6, 8]

False positives can occur

> Because reactive and malignant adenopathy are often radiographically indistinguishable unless there is a benign pattern of calcification

Conventional Tomography

Examination of choice for hilar evaluation if patient is a healthy adult nonsmoker and there is only marginal radiographic evidence of isolated unilateral hilar enlargement on chest radiographs

Can supplement CT in planning tracheobronchial surgery because it demonstrates the overall architecture of the tracheobronchial tree more concisely than CT, in a format that, as yet, may be more familiar to nonradiologists

Sensitivity

For detecting malignant hilar adenopathy: average *78%* [4, 8]

For detecting malignant mediastinal adenopathy: *61%* [5, 6, 8]

False negatives can occur because

> Adjacent vascular structures are complex

> Early malignant adenopathy may not enlarge hilar lymph nodes

Adenopathy lying medial to vessels may not produce an abnormal hilar contour

Specificity

For indicating normal hila in patients with lung cancer: average 71% [4, 8]
For indicating normal mediastinum in patients with lung cancer: average 91% [5, 6, 8]
False positives can occur
> Because reactive and malignant adenopathy are often radiographically indistinguishable unless there is a benign pattern of calcification
> If vascular abnormalities, particularly when asymmetric, simulate adenopathy
> If supine positioning and complex motion tomography cause normal or dilated vessels to simulate hilar adenopathy

Contribution of Magnetic Resonance Imaging [1, 7, 9, 10]

Potentially excellent method of distinguishing enlarged pulmonary vessels from hilar nodes, and showing the relationship of hilar masses to mediastinal masses without contrast agent

References

1. Berquist, T. H., Brown, L. R., and May, G. R. Magnetic resonance imaging of the chest: A diagnostic comparison with computed tomography and hilar tomography. *Magnetic Resonance Imaging* 2:315, 1984.
2. Broderick, T. W. Contrast Material Reactions. In G. W. Friedland, R. Filly, and M. L. Goris (Eds.). *Uroradiology.* New York: Churchill Livingstone, 1983.
3. Faling, L. J., Pugatch, R. D., Jung-Legg, Y., et al. Computed tomographic scanning of the mediastinum in the staging of bronchogenic carcinoma. *Am. Rev. Respir. Dis.* 124:690, 1981.
4. Glazer, G. M., Francis, I. R., Shirazi, K. K., et al. Evaluation of the pulmonary hilum: Comparison of conventional radiography, 55° posterior oblique tomography, and dynamic computed tomography. *J. Comput. Assist. Tomogr.* 7:983, 1983.
5. Hirleman, M. T., Yie-Chiu, V. S., Chiu, L. C., et al. The resectability of primary lung carcinoma: A diagnostic staging review. *J. Comput. Assist. Tomogr.* 4:146, 1980.
6. Lewis, J. R., Jr., Madrazo, B. L., Gross, S. C., et al. The value of radiographic and computed tomography in the staging of lung carcinoma. *Ann. Thoracic Surg.* 34:553, 1982.
7. O'Donovan, P. B., Ross, J. S., Sivak, E. D., et al. Magnetic resonance imaging of the thorax: The advantages of coronal and saggital planes. *AJR* 143:1183, 1984.
8. Osborne, D. R., Korobkin, M., Ravin, C. E., et al. Comparison of plain radiography, conventional tomography, and computed to-

mography in detecting intrathoracic lymph node metastases from lung carcinoma. *Radiology* 142:157, 1982.

9. Webb, W. R., Gamsu, G., Stark, D. D., et al. Magnetic resonance imaging of the normal and abnormal pulmonary hila. *Radiology* 152:89, 1984.

10. Webb, W. R., Jensen, B. G., Gamsu, G., et al. Coronal magnetic resonance imaging of the chest: Normal and abnormal. *Radiology* 153:729, 1984.

11. Winterbauer, R. H., Belic, N., and Moores, K. D. A clinical interpretation of bilateral hilar adenopathy. *Ann. Intern. Med.* 78:65, 1973.

Diagnosis of Pulmonary Embolism

Barbara J. McNeil

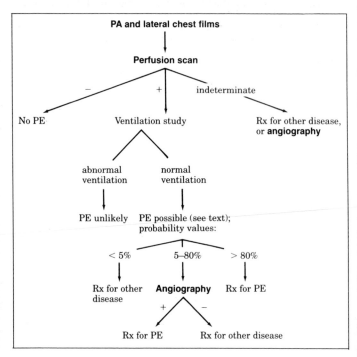

Typical Patient

Individual with chest pain, shortness of breath, venous disease, hemoptysis, or syncope, suspected of having pulmonary embolism

Typical Disorder(s)

Recent pulmonary embolism, pneumonia, asthma, chronic lung disease, bronchogenic carcinoma, "pleurodynia"

Comments

This algorithm does not discuss the value of blood gases in the diagnosis of pulmonary embolism because of their poor sensitivity and specificity; nor does it discuss digital subtraction angiography because of its low sensitivity (less than 80%) [4]

Plain Chest Film

Identifies abnormal areas that may either explain initial symptoms or that may complicate reading of lung scan
Essential for interpreting lung scan

Drawbacks

Insensitive and nonspecific

Sensitivity

Considering any of the findings thought "characteristic of pulmonary embolism" (e.g., elevated hemidiaphragm, relative hypovolemia, pleural effusion): *33%* [7]

Specificity

80% [7]

Technetium-99m Macroaggregated Albumin (MAA) Perfusion Lung Scan

Identifies abnormalities in regional perfusion but must be coupled with ventilation study to increase specificity
Trapping particles in precapillary arterioles coupled with low energy of technetium make examination safe in pregnant women

Drawbacks

Any of a wide variety of processes will lead to alterations in perfusion
About 35% of patients with pulmonary emboli never completely resolve their perfusion abnormalities, thus making it difficult to differentiate new from old emboli
Sensitivity and specificity decrease in patients with very severe COPD [1]

Sensitivity-Specificity Relationships

By considering *any* perfusion abnormality suspect for pulmonary embolism sensitivity is *100%* [5]
Otherwise, sensitivity and specificity vary markedly with the ventilation-perfusion observed: size and number of perfusion defects, associated radiographic abnormalities, and presence or absence of normal ($\dot{V}/\dot{Q}$ mismatch) or abnormal ($\dot{V}/\dot{Q}$ match) ventilation in areas of abnormal perfusion
When the scan findings match in size and location the radiographic abnormalities, the scan is called *indeterminate,* and the probability of pulmonary embolism after the scan is the same as it was before the scan [3]
For the diagnosis of pulmonary emboli, data on sensitivity and specificity are usually combined (using Bayes' theorem) with a previous estimate of risk in a given patient to give probabil-

Table 25-1. Probability Estimates for Pulmonary Embolism Associated with Common Scan Patterns in Three Clinical Situations

	Clinical Situation		
Scan Pattern	Low Risk	Average Risk	High Risk
Single perfusion defect, corresponding to chest film abnormality ("indeterminate pattern")	.05	.15	.55
Multiple defects, segmental or lobar in size			
No ventilation study	.13	.35	.79
$\dot{V}/\dot{Q}$ mismatch	.54	.80	.96
$\dot{V}/\dot{Q}$ match	*	*	*
Multiple defects, subsegmental only in size			
No ventilation study	.005	.02	.11
$\dot{V}/\dot{Q}$ mismatch	.01	.04	.20
$\dot{V}/\dot{Q}$ match	*	*	*

*In general, data from most studies indicate that these patients have a very low (close to zero) chance of having pulmonary embolism; however, one Canadian study has indicated that 3 of 13 patients with $\dot{V}/\dot{Q}$ matches may have pulmonary embolism [8]

ity estimates for the presence of pulmonary emboli [1, 2, 10] (Table 25-1)

False positive perfusion studies can occur from
    Anything that leads to increased vascular resistance (e.g., congestive heart failure, pneumonia)
    Alveolar hypoxia and reflex vasoconstriction
    Extrinsic compression of pulmonary vasculature
    Nonvascular thrombi (fat, tumor, or amniotic fluid emboli)
    Bronchopulmonary anastomoses

False positive ventilation-perfusion studies (i.e., $\dot{V}/\dot{Q}$ mismatch but no pulmonary embolism) can occur from [9]
    Old pulmonary emboli
    Any form of vasculitis or any abnormality (e.g., multiple congenital stenoses) of pulmonary vessels
    Lymphangitic carcinomatosis
    Intravenous drug abuse
    Radiation therapy
    Early pneumonia
    Pulmonary hypertension
    Bronchogenic carcinoma

False negative ventilation-perfusion studies (i.e., $\dot{V}/\dot{Q}$ match but pulmonary embolism) can occur
    Very early (minutes) after embolic event

In patients with severe COPD
Rarely in acute pulmonary embolism [8]

Pulmonary Angiography

Invasive, but currently considered the gold standard for diagnosis of pulmonary embolism, particularly with magnification views and superselective injections [6, 13]
Visualizes embolus directly rather than reflecting the probable cause of symptoms, as do peripheral venography and impedance plethysmography [11]
With experience and calibration interobserver variation in interpretation is less than 3% [6]
Allows simultaneous hemodynamic assessment

Disadvantages

Complications: total 4%, including arrhythmias and rarely perforation of right ventricle; mortality, .3% [6]; higher complication rates among patients with pulmonary hypertension
  Institutions rarely performing angiography will probably have a higher complication rate
Should be done with caution in individuals with severe congestive heart failure

Sensitivity

By definition as gold standard, extremely high if performed shortly after acute event
Considerably higher than peripheral venography or impedance plethysmography; about *30%* of patients will have positive pulmonary angiograms and negative studies of peripheral system [8]
False negatives can occur if
  Angiography is performed late after embolic event—at this time either no signs or only secondary nonspecific signs of embolization may be present
  Inappropriate vessel is injected
  Study is inadequate (e.g., oblique views may be required but not obtained)
  Compositive vascular and airway shadows are misinterpreted

Specificity

With rigid criteria for assessment (viewing the cut-off vessel, trailing end of clot, or defect of clot), considered to be *100%*
False positives can occur if
  Rigid criteria are not used for interpretation and hence old emboli are confused with new

Contribution of Magnetic Resonance Imaging [12, 15]

Visualizes blood vessels without contrast agent
Visualizes large central thrombi, but MRI's role in defining more
peripheral emboli remains uncertain

References

1. Alderson, P. O., Biello, D. R., Sachariah, K. G., et al. Scintigraphic detection of pulmonary embolism in patients with obstructive pulmonary disease. *Radiology* 138:661, 1981.
2. Biello, D. R., Mattar, A. G., McKnight, R. C., et al. Ventilation-perfusion studies in suspected pulmonary embolism. *AJR* 133:1033, 1979.
3. Biello, D. R., Mattar, A. G., Osei-Wusu, A., et al. Interpretation of indeterminate lung scintigrams. *Radiology* 133:189, 1979.
4. Ferris, E. J., Holder, J. C., Lim, W. N., et al. Angiography of pulmonary emboli: Digital studies and balloon occlusion cineangiography. *AJR* 142:369, 1984.
5. Greenspan, R. H. Does a normal isotope perfusion scan exclude pulmonary embolism? *Invest. Radiol.* 8:97, 1973.
6. Greenspan, R. H. Angiography in Pulmonary Embolism. In H. L. Abrams (Ed.). *Abrams Angiography: Vascular and Interventional Radiology* (3rd ed.). Boston: Little, Brown, 1983. Pp. 803–816.
7. Greenspan, R. H., Ravin, C. E., Polansky, S. M., et al. Accuracy of the chest radiograph in diagnosis of pulmonary embolism. *Invest. Radiol.* 17:539, 1982.
8. Hull, R. D., Hirsch, J., Carter, C. J., et al. Pulmonary angiography, ventilation lung scanning, and venography for clinically suspected pulmonary embolism with abnormal perfusion lung scan. *Ann. Intern. Med.* 98:891, 1983.
9. Li, D. K., Seltzer, S. S., and McNeil, B. J. V/Q mismatches unassociated with pulmonary embolism: Case report and review of the literature. *J. Nucl. Med.* 19:1331, 1978.
10. McNeil, B. J. Ventilation-perfusion studies and the diagnosis of pulmonary embolism: Concise communication. *J. Nucl. Med.* 21:319, 1980.
11. Mohr, D. N. Venous thrombosis and pulmonary embolism: Their relationship and its importance in the evaluation of patients with suspected pulmonary embolism. *Cardiovasc. Rev. Rep.* 5:936, 1984.
12. Moore, E. H., Gamsu, G., Webb, W. R., et al. Pulmonary embolus: Detection and follow-up using magnetic resonance. *Radiology* 153:471, 1984.
13. Novelline, R. A., Baltarowich, O. H., Athanasoulis, C. A., et al. The clinical course of patients with suspected pulmonary embolism and a negative pulmonary arteriogram. *Radiology* 126:561, 1978.
14. Sasahara, A. A., Hyers, T. M., Cole, C. M., et al. The urokinase pulmonary embolism trial. A national cooperative study. *Circulation* 47(Suppl. II):1, 1973.
15. Thickman, D., Kressel, H. Y., and Axel, L. Demonstration of pulmonary embolism by magnetic resonance imaging. *AJR* 142:921, 1984.

Solitary Pulmonary Nodule (<3 cm)

Robert D. Pugatch

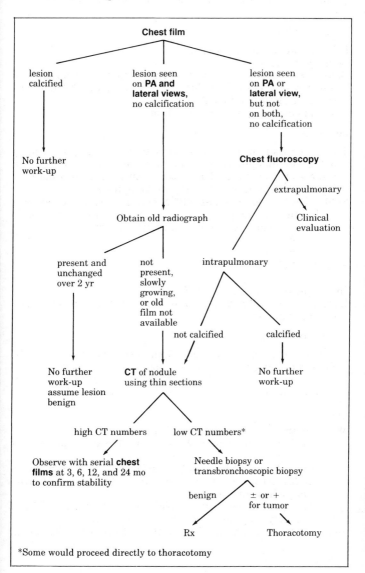

*Some would proceed directly to thoracotomy

Typical Patient

Individual having a 3 cm or less homogeneous parenchymal lesion with sharply defined margins, typically revealed on a chest radiograph

Typical Disorder(s)

Primary bronchogenic carcinoma
Solitary metastasis
Benign nonneoplastic processes: granulomas, intrapulmonary bronchogenic cysts, bronchial atresia, traumatic hematomas, vascular abnormalities (AVMs)
Benign neoplasms: hamartomas, bronchial adenomas

Comments

The major issue in this situation is characterizing a lesion as benign or malignant. The only accepted criteria for benign disease are: no growth demonstrated on serial chest films over 2 years or calcification in a typical benign pattern
Solitary pulmonary nodules (SPNs) may be the manifestation of early lung cancer: 40% of 1200 lung cancers were originally detected as peripheral pulmonary mass lesions [8]

Plain Chest Film

Initial means of detecting all SPNs
Evaluates the status of the hilum and mediastinum when lung cancer is known

Drawbacks

Detection threshold is generally 1 cm; lesions of 1–2 cm can be missed because of overlapping bony thorax or blood vessels
Lesions less than 1 cm wide are often missed; retrospective reviews show a high incidence of misses on prior films

Comments

Where extrathoracic malignancy is known
    Osteogenic sarcoma: SPN is almost always a metastasis (95%)
    Breast, kidney: SPN will be a primary lung cancer almost half the time among smokers unless breast or renal cancer is disseminated
    Primary head/neck tumor: With localized tumor, SPN is a primary lung cancer in up to 90% of cases
In a nonsmoker less than 35 years of age, SPN is usually benign

Sensitivity

Because initially all SPNs are detected by chest films, sensitivity is by definition high

False negatives can occur

> For detection: by failing to recognize nodule because of overlapping bony thorax or blood vessels
>
> For diagnosis: by misinterpreting the presence and/or pattern of calcification
>
> For diagnosis: by not aggressively pursuing a tissue diagnosis

Specificity

With specific patterns of calcification: a benign SPN is assured (e.g., eccentric calcification may represent cancer engulfing a pre-existing granuloma)

For a noncalcified nodule: variable according to population

False positives can occur

> If an extraparenchymal lesion is mistaken for a parenchymal abnormality

Chest Fluoroscopy

Can detect calcification in some benign nodules
Distinguishes some nodules from overlapping structures
Interactive examination permits precise localization of lesions
Patient maneuvers must be undertaken under direct vision of radiologist

Drawbacks

Relatively poor resolution restricts utility to relatively large lesions

Sensitivity and Specificity

False negatives and *false positives* can occur

> With an inexperienced operator

Computed Tomography (CT)

Accurately detects and characterizes calcification within nodule
Confirms presence of nodule with certainty
Detects "occult" lesions elsewhere and provides information about regional lymph node involvement

Drawbacks

Specificity for small noncalcified lesion overlooked on chest radiography or tomography (3 mm to 1.0 cm range) is unknown

Waiting time for study may be long

Rare complications; occasional contrast reactions and/or secondary renal failure occur, but serious reactions only 1 in 14,000 [1]

Comments

Examination should be preceded by a chest film to detect and locate the abnormality

There is still some controversy over the relative benefit of CT in this situation: Some observers have found that chest films or conventional tomography generally demonstrate the calcification of lesions shown to be calcified on CT [3]

Sensitivity

For detecting SPNs: extremely high, highest of all current imaging modalities

False negatives can occur if

Lesion size is not above threshold of resolution

Lesion is not visualized because of partial volume effects or variation in patient respiration

Specificity

For differentiating benign from malignant

If (high) CT numbers indicate calcification: very high [3, 5]

If CT numbers do not show calcification: variable; about 50% of benign lesions and most malignant lesions will have low CT numbers [3, 5]

False positives can occur

If benign lesion does not contain calcification or it is not recognized, i.e., calling benign lesions malignant

References

1. Broderick, T. W. Contrast Material Reactions. In G. W. Friedland, R. Filly, and M. L. Goris (Eds.). *Uroradiology.* New York: Churchill Livingstone, 1983.
2. Fraser, R. G., and Paré, J. A. P. *Diagnosis of Diseases of the Chest* (2nd ed.). Philadelphia: Saunders, 1979. Vol. 4, pp. 2181–2190.
3. Godwin, J. D., Speckman, J. M., Fram, E. K., et al. Distinguishing benign from malignant pulmonary nodules by computed tomography. *Radiology* 144:349, 1982.
4. Muhm, J. R., Miller, W. E., Fontana, R. S., et al. Lung cancer detected during a screening program using four-month chest radiographs. *Radiology* 148:609, 1983.
5. Siegelman, S. S., Zerhouni, E. A., Leo, F. P., et al. CT of the solitary pulmonary nodule. *AJR* 135:1, 1980.

6. Steele, J. D., Kleitsch, W. P., Dunn, J. E., Jr., et al. Survival in males with bronchogenic carcinomas resected as asymptomatic solitary pulmonary nodules. *Ann. Thorac. Surg.* 2:368, 1966.
7. Stitik, F. P., and Tockman, M. S. Radiographic screening in the early detection of lung cancer. *Radiol. Clin. North Am.* 16:347, 1978.
8. Theros, E. G. 1976 Caldwell Lecture. Varying manifestations of peripheral pulmonary neoplasms: A radiologic-pathologic correlative study. *AJR* 128:893, 1977.

Neurological Disease

Asymptomatic Carotid Bruit

Daniel H. O'Leary

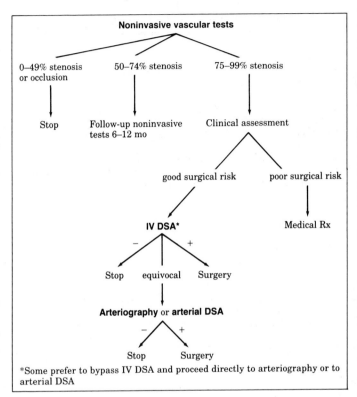

Noninvasive vascular tests

0–49% stenosis or occlusion → Stop

50–74% stenosis → Follow-up noninvasive tests 6–12 mo

75–99% stenosis → Clinical assessment

Clinical assessment → good surgical risk / poor surgical risk

poor surgical risk → Medical Rx

good surgical risk → **IV DSA***

IV DSA − → Stop
equivocal
IV DSA + → Surgery

equivocal → **Arteriography** or **arterial DSA**

Arteriography − → Stop
Arteriography + → Surgery

*Some prefer to bypass IV DSA and proceed directly to arteriography or to arterial DSA

Typical Patient

Individual with bruit and without localizing hemispheric symptoms

Typical Disorder(s)

Atherosclerotic plaque or stenosis in common carotid artery or major branches
Normal vessel

Comments

Asymptomatic bruits are a risk factor for stroke [12, 22]; with carotid stenosis of greater than 75%, the risk is significantly higher than for those with bruits and stenosis of 0–49% [5]
75% of strokes occur in the carotid circulation [14]
90% of strokes occur without prior transient ischemic attacks [21]

The majority of patients with bruits will have a 50% or greater stenosis [10]

The efficacy of carotid endarterectomy for asymptomatic patients remains controversial [5]

The presence of a carotid bruit is a better indicator of systemic atherosclerotic disease than of impending stroke [12, 22]

Noninvasive Vascular Tests (Sonography— B-scan and Doppler)

Highly accurate in detecting stenosis of 50% or greater

Provides both anatomical and physiological data

Adequate examination achieved in all but a few percent of patients

Serial examinations may be used to follow patients over time

Because patients are asymptomatic, if examination is normal, no further evaluation is necessary [16]

Drawbacks

Results are not self-explanatory to referring physician

Cannot detect intracranial abnormalities

Does not visualize the aortic arch

Cannot reliably identify ulceration [13, 23, 25]

May confuse external with internal carotid stenosis

May overdiagnose occlusion

May not be able to distinguish between near-total occlusion and total occlusion [18, 23]

Positive results generally require a second examination (angiography) be performed before treatment

May be overused and lead to unnecessary angiography and surgery

Comments

The use of oculoplethysmography will reduce the number of noninvasive false positive tests by compensating for the tendency for ultrasound to overdiagnose occlusion and to mistake external for internal carotid stenosis

Sensitivity

Averages greater than 90%, with a range of 85–95% [2–4, 7, 8, 13, 18–20, 23, 25]

False negatives can occur with
   Minimally echogenic plaques
   Total occlusions
   Shadowing of the lesion secondary to calcium
   Intracranial stenoses

Specificity

Averages greater than 90%, with a range of 80–95% [2–4, 7, 8, 13, 18–20, 23, 25]

False positives occur with
> Kinking of the proximal internal carotid
> External carotid stenosis

Intravenous Digital Subtraction Angiography (IV DSA)

May serve as a definitive study
Less operator dependent than ultrasound
Can be performed on an outpatient basis
Image format is easily understood by physicians
Visualizes aortic arch and carotid siphon

Drawbacks

15–30% of examinations are nondiagnostic [6, 9]
May require using large volume of contrast
Less risk than angiography, but more contrast reactions may occur

Sensitivity

For detecting stenosis of more than 40% of internal carotid artery: at least *85%* [15], sometimes reported as high as *93%* [24]
False negatives can occur
> If carotids are not well visualized (sensitivity may drop to *54%*) [6]

Specificity

Greater than *90%* [6, 15]
False positives can occur
> If carotids are not well visualized (specificity may drop to *70%*) [6]

Arteriography

Definitive study
Identifies intracranial abnormalities
Results are easily understood by referring physician

Drawbacks

Complications: Contrast reaction and/or secondary renal failure, rare; vascular injury and thrombosis, serious, about 1%; local hemorrhage or hematoma, nonfatal serious reactions, less than 2%; fatalities, .03% [11]

Sensitivity

For definition of flow reducing lesions: high

Specificity

High

Arterial Digital Subtraction Angiography (DSA)

Definitive study
Image quality comparable to standard angiography
Identifies intracranial abnormalities
Image format familiar to physician
May be performed on an outpatient basis

Drawbacks

Invasive, with risk factors not yet definitely established, although probably safer than standard angiography

Comments

The combination of prescreening of patients by noninvasive tests followed by outpatient arterial DSA studies with No. 4 French catheters in appropriate instances may be the most efficacious manner by which to evaluate patients with suspected cerebral vascular disease

Sensitivity

No data available, but presumably similar to conventional arteriography

Specificity

No data available, but presumably similar to conventional arteriography

Contribution of Magnetic Resonance Imaging [17]

May represent an excellent noninvasive approach to arteriosclerotic plaques and abnormal flow patterns

References

1. Aaron, J. O., Hesselink, J. R., Oat, R., et al. Complication of intravenous DSA performed for carotid artery disease: A prospective study. *Radiology* 153:675, 1984.
2. Ackerman, R. H. Noninvasive carotid evaluation. *Stroke* 11:675, 1980.
3. Blackshear, W. M., Phillips, D. J., Thiele, B. L., et al. Detection of carotid occlusive disease by ultrasonic imaging and pulsed Doppler spectrum analysis. *Surgery* 86:698, 1979.
4. Cape, C. A., DeSaussure, R. L., and Nixon, J. Carotid ultrasonography in carotid artery disease. *South. Med. J.* 77:183, 1984.
5. Chambers, B. R., and Norris, J. W. The case against surgery for asymptomatic carotid stenosis. *Stroke* 15:964, 1984.
6. Chilcote, W. A., Modic, M. T., Pavlicek, W. A., et al. Digital subtraction angiography of the carotid arteries: A comparative study in 100 patients. *Radiology* 139:287, 1981.

7. Comerota, A. J., Cranley, J. J., Katz, M. L., et al. Real-time B-mode carotid imaging. *J. Vasc. Surg.* 1:84, 1984.
8. Crummy, A. B., Zweibel, W. J., Barriga, P., et al. Doppler evaluation of extracranial cerebrovascular disease. *AJR* 132:91, 1979.
9. Foley, W. D., Smith, D. F., Milde, M. W., et al. Intravenous DSA examination of patients with suspected cerebral ischemia. *Radiology* 151:651, 1984.
10. Hennerici, M., Aublich, A., Sandmann, W., et al. Incidence of asymptomatic extracranial arterial disease. *Stroke* 12:750, 1981.
11. Hessel, S. J. Complications of Angiography and Other Catheter Procedures. In H. L. Abrams (Ed.). *Abrams Angiography: Vascular and Interventional Radiology* (3rd ed.). Boston: Little, Brown, 1983. Pp. 1041–1055.
12. Heyman, A., Wilkinson, W. E., Heyden, S., et al. Risk of stroke in asymptomatic persons with cervical arterial bruits. *N. Engl. J. Med.* 302:838, 1980.
13. James, E. M., Earnest, F., Forbes, G. S., et al. High-resolution dynamic ultrasound imaging of the carotid bifurcation: A prospective evaluation. *Radiology* 144:853, 1982.
14. Kuller, L. H., and Sutton, K. C. Carotid artery bruit and neck auscultation. *Stroke* 15:944, 1984.
15. Kempczinski, R. F., Wood, G. W., Berlatzky, Y,., et al. A comparison of digital subtraction angiography and noninvasive testing in the diagnosis of cerebrovascular disease. *Am. J. Surg.* 146:203, 1983.
16. Long, J. B., Lynch, T. G., Karanfilian, R. G., et al. Asymptomatic carotid disease. *Surg. Gynecol. Obstet.* 160:89, 1985.
17. Mills, C. M., Brant-Zawadzki, M., Crooks, L. E., et al. Nuclear magnetic resonance: Principles of blood flow imaging. *AJR* 142:165, 1984.
18. O'Leary, D. H., Gibbons, G. W., and Pinel, D. F. Limitations of noninvasive testing in assessing the "occluded" carotid artery. *AJNR* 4:759, 1983.
19. O'Leary, D. H., Persson, A. V., and Clouse, M. E. Noninvasive testing for carotid artery stenosis. *AJNR* 2:437, 1981; *AJR* 137:1189, 1981.
20. Wetzner, S. M., Kiser, L. C., and Bezrek, J. S. Duplex ultrasound imaging: Vascular applications. *Radiology* 150:507, 1984.
21. Whisnant, J. P. The role of the neurologist in the decline of stroke. *Ann. Neurol.* 14:1, 1983.
22. Wolf, P. A., Kannel, W. B., Sorlie, P., et al. Asymptomatic carotid bruit and risk of stroke—the Framingham study. *JAMA* 245:1442, 1981.
23. Wolverson, M. K., Herberg, E., Sundaram, M., et al. Carotid atherosclerosis: High-resolution real-time sonography correlated with angiography. *AJNR* 3:601, 1982.
24. Wood, G. W., Lukin, R. R., Tomsick, T. A., et al. Digital subtraction angiography with intravenous injection: Assessment of 1000 carotid bifurcations. *AJR* 140:855, 1983.
25. Zwiebel, W. J., Austin, C. W., Sackett, J. F., et al. Correlation of high-resolution, B-mode and continuous-wave Doppler sonography with arteriography in the diagnosis of carotid stenosis. *Radiology* 149:523, 1983.

Management of Transient Ischemic Attacks

H. Harris Funkenstein

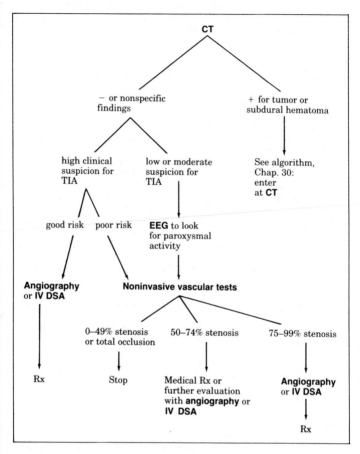

Typical Patient

Individual experiencing transient (minutes to hours) focal neurological symptoms. A typical transient ischemic attack may consist of symptoms related to either the carotid or the basilar territory.

If carotid territory is involved, symptoms may consist of:

  Brief loss of vision, either of a sector of vision or "like a curtain coming down"

  Tingling or numbness on one side of the face or one extremity

  Weakness or clumsiness of a limb or of one side

  Slurred or aphasic speech

If vertebrobasilar territory is involved, symptoms may consist
of:
  Unsteady gait, falling to one side
  Weakness of one or more limbs, sometimes bilateral
  Tingling or numbness of one or more limbs
  Visual blurring, diplopia
  Numbness of the face
  Dssarthria, difficulty swallowing
If symptoms persist or relevant neurological findings are seen
on examination at 24 hours, then a stroke has occurred

Typical Disorder(s)

Atherosclerotic narrowing of extracranial or intracranial vessel
Atherosclerotic plaque at origin of internal carotid artery
Embolus to cortical branch of cerebral artery
In addition to these disorders, the differential diagnosis of such
transient symptoms includes:
  Vestibulopathy
  Migraine
  Focal seizures

Head Computed Tomography (CT)

Documents presence of stroke or prior strokes
Useful in excluding conditions (tumor, subdural hematoma, arteriovenous malformation) that may produce transient neurological symptoms

Comments

Useful in recognizing recent infarcts that might contraindicate
early endarterectomy save for the recent stroke
Required before anticoagulation to reduce risk of bleeding

Drawbacks

In transient ischemic attacks CT is either negative or shows
nonrelevant abnormality

Sensitivity

For tumors, subdural hematomas, arteriovenous malformations: high (see Chap. 30, p. 155)

Specificity

In general, for most categories of patients: high (see Chap. 30,
p. 155)

Electroencephalography (EEG)

Useful in recognizing focal seizures by the presence of focal
sharp activity or spikes

May be useful in recognizing the occurrence of a small cortical stroke by the presence of focal slowing

Drawbacks

Not helpful if small stroke spares cortical structures (e.g., in brainstem strokes)

Sensitivity

High if stroke affects cortical structures and occurred within several days; declines as site of injury moves from cortex to white matter and deep nuclei
False negatives can occur
    Even in clear cases of focal seizures

Specificity

For showing normal cortex: high
For determining causes of abnormalities: low

Noninvasive Vascular Tests (Sonography— B-scan and Doppler)

Indicates if significant carotid stenosis or occlusion exists
Indicates if carotid bifurcation is involved by atherosclerosis (and hence possible source of embolic material)

Drawbacks

May not distinguish between high-grade stenosis (patient still at risk) and complete occlusion (patient at lower risk) [7, 8]
May not distinguish between uncomplicated atheromatous narrowing and ulcerated plaque [9]

Comments

Useful screening test where picture is unclear, especially if patient is not candidate for anticoagulation for intracranial disease
Hemodynamically significant lesions compromise 85% of the cross-sectional luminal area or reduce the carotid diameter to 1 mm or less
If degree of stenosis is 70–85% on Doppler or B-scan, indirect tests of carotid circulation (orbital Doppler, thermography, oculoplethysmography) may prove helpful

Sensitivity

Recognition of significant carotid stenosis in *85–95%* of cases [1]
False negatives can occur with
    Shadowing secondary to heavy calcium deposits
    Very low flow secondary to total occlusion
    Intracranial stenoses

Specificity

Ranges from *85–95%* [1]
False positives can occur
    With extremely tortuous vessels or external carotid stenosis

Selective Cerebral Angiography

High reliability in recognizing stenosis and/or occlusion of both extracranial and intracranial vessels
Higher reliability in recognizing carotid ulcerations than digital subtraction angiography
Provides information about collateral circulation
Documents presence of tumors, arteriovenous malformations, and subdural hematomas

Drawbacks

Complications—stroke, myocardial infarction, arrhythmia, occlusion of vessel, local hematoma, confusion, transient neurological deficits—in 2–25% of patients studied depending on center and vessels catheterized [3, 5]
Dye reactions and/or secondary renal failure rarely
Fatalities in 0.03–0.1%—usually myocardial infarction or major stroke
Delays anticoagulation by time required for arteriotomy to seal (8–12 hours)

Sensitivity

For recognition of significant stenoses, either extracranial or intracranial: greater than *90%*
For recognition of ulcerated plaques: *50–75%*

Specificity

For significant stenoses: approaching *100%*

Intravenous Digital Subtraction Angiography (IV DSA)

Useful in documenting carotid narrowing at common or internal carotid level
May be useful in recognizing stenosis of the carotid siphon, though much less likely

Drawbacks

Requires cooperative patient with adequate cardiac output
15–30% of examinations may produce inadequate visualization [4]
Dye load may be hazardous in patients with compromised renal function
Usually misses stenosis of proximal intracranial vessels

Comments

Morbidity/mortality less than selective angiography (about 0.5%)

Imaging of posterior circulation is difficult; only major vessels are visualized, and then variably

Sensitivity

Depends on adequacy of visualization

For studies with adequate visualization, carotid stenosis of greater than 50% is recognized in *80–90%* of investigations; for all studies sensitivity drops to *50–60%* [2]

Specificity

Greater than *85–90%*

False positives increase as quality of visualization diminishes (specificity drops to *70%* overall) [2]

Contribution of Magnetic Resonance Imaging [6]

May represent an excellent noninvasive approach to arteriosclerotic plaques and abnormal flow patterns

References

1. Ackerman, R. H. Noninvasive carotid evaluation. *Stroke* 11:675, 1980.
2. Chilcote, W. A., Modic, M. T., Pavlicek, W. A., et al. Digital subtraction angiography of the carotid arteries: A comparative study in 100 patients. *Radiology* 139:287, 1981.
3. Faught, E., Trader, S. D., and Hanna, G. R. Cerebral complications of angiography for transient ischemia and stroke: Prediction of risk. *Neurology* 29:4, 1979.
4. Foley, W. D., Smith, D. F., Milde, M. W., et al. Intravenous DSA examination of patients with suspected cerebral ischemia. *Radiology* 151:651, 1984.
5. Hass, W. K., Fields, W. S., North, R. R., et al. Joint study of extracranial arterial occlusion. II. Arteriography techniques, sites and complications. *JAMA* 203:961, 1968.
6. Mills, C. M., Brant-Zawadzki, M., Crooks, L. E., et al. Nuclear magnetic resonance: Principles of blood flow imaging. *AJR* 142:165, 1984.
7. O'Leary, D. H., Gibbons, G. W., Pinel, D. F. Limitations of noninvasive testing in assessing the "occluded" carotid artery. *AJNR* 4:759, 1983.
8. Wolverson, M. K., Heiberg, E., Sundaram, E., et al. Carotid atherosclerosis: High resolution real-time sonography correlated with angiography. *AJR* 140:355, 1983.
9. Zwiebel, W. J., Austin, C. W., Sackett, J. F., et al. Correlation of high-resolution, B-mode and continuous-wave Doppler sonography with arteriography in the diagnosis of carotid stenosis. *Radiology* 149:523, 1983.

Management of Stroke

H. Harris Funkenstein

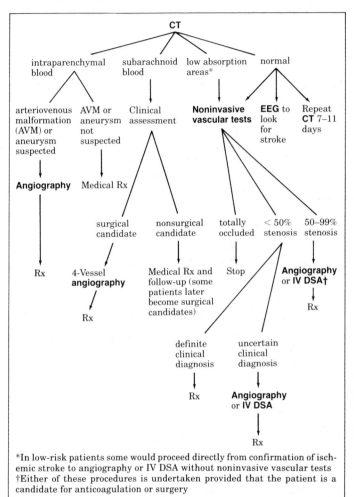

*In low-risk patients some would proceed directly from confirmation of ischemic stroke to angiography or IV DSA without noninvasive vascular tests
†Either of these procedures is undertaken provided that the patient is a candidate for anticoagulation or surgery

Typical Patient

Individual experiencing persistent (greater than 24 hours) focal neurological symptoms and/or signs of acute onset (over minutes or a few hours). Patients with symptoms lasting several hours but not yet 24 hours should be considered to have a probable stroke. Deficits seen may include:

Impaired consciousness

Monoparesis or hemiparesis
Sensory deficits (tingling, numbness)
Dysarthria, dysphasia
Diplopia
Visual field defects
Ataxia of limbs or trunk
Others depending on site of lesion

Typical Disorder(s) [11, 12]

Infarction in carotid or vertebrobasilar territory secondary to thrombosis of a major vessel

Infarction secondary to thrombosis of a small vessel (lacune or basilar branch disease)

Embolism of a small or large vessel

Intraparenchymal hemorrhage secondary to hypertension, coagulopathy, trauma, vascular anomaly

Subarachnoid hemorrhage secondary to arteriovenous malformation or aneurysm

Head Computed Tomography (CT)

Recognizes presence of hemorrhage

Indicates presence of hemorrhagic infarction by presence of irregular area of blood density associated with infarct

Indicates presence and location of infarction by showing low-density region

Indicates presence of other lesion (subdural hematoma, tumor, abscess) in patient thought to have stroke

Recognizes larger aneurysms (greater than 1.0–1.5 cm diameter) and arteriovenous malformation

Demonstrates subarachnoid blood in major subarachnoid hemorrhages

Drawbacks

May not distinguish hemorrhage from hemorrhagic infarction in all cases

May miss small strokes, especially those secondary to small vessel occlusion, or early strokes (within 24 hours) [3, 6]

Comments

Early missed strokes may be diagnosed by repeat CT scans at 7–14 days

Presence of hemorrhagic infarction is one criterion for delaying anticoagulation in patients with infarction

Not infrequently (in 10–20% of patients) infarctions may enhance with contrast and the distinction between stroke and tumor be unclear; this rarely occurs within the first 7 days after infarction; repeat CT may be helpful [16]

Aneurysms may be recognized on contrast-enhanced CT scans provided they exceed 0.5–1.0 cm in diameter

Small subarachnoid hemorrhages may escape detection on CT; lumbar puncture is diagnostic

Arteriovenous malformations (AVM) will be recognized in almost 100% of cases if contrast is used; occasionally differential between hemorrhagic infarction and AVM will depend on the clinical picture or the results of arteriography

Sensitivity

For bland infarcts: *50–75%*

False negatives can occur and usually reflect:

      Small size of infarct (lacune)

      Brain stem location

      Timing of CT (most sensitive at 8–11 days)

For intraparenchymal hemorrhage: approaches *100%* (limited only by adequacy of study)

For subarachnoid hemorrhages within several days with impaired consciousness: high

For all subarachnoid hemorrhages: at least *70%* [10, 17]

For aneurysms greater than 1.0 cm: high if contrast used

For arteriovenous malformations: near *100%* if contrast used

Specificity

In general, high for most categories of patients: greater than *95%*

Rarely, *false positives* may occur with tumors or demyelinating plaques

Noninvasive Vascular Tests (B-scan and Doppler)

Documents presence of complete stenosis (as etiology of stroke) or marked stenosis (possibly incomplete stroke)

Less frequently recognizes ulcerated plaque as source of small embolus [8, 18]

Drawbacks

May not distinguish complete occlusion of carotid from severe stenosis [14]

Fails to address problems of intracranial circulation

Sensitivity

For carotid occlusion: *85–95%* [2, 15], but may fail to distinguish complete occlusion from severe stenosis

For carotid ulceration: low

Specificity

For carotid occlusion: very high (*80–95%*) [2, 15]

For carotid ulceration: low

Electroencephalography (EEG)

Provides evidence for small vessel disease in that EEG may be
normal or show only diffuse slowing

Comments

Strokes involving cortex or underlying white matter usually
produce focal abnormalities, especially within first few weeks
[1]

Cerebral Angiography

Diagnoses nature of vascular pathology in ischemic stroke

Delineates presence and amount of collateral circulation to infarcted area

May provide evidence for infarction in the form of luxury perfusion and early draining veins

Demonstrates major vessel stenoses that may result in distal
emboli

Demonstrates other vascular changes such as fibromuscular
dysplasia, dissection of carotid, or vasculitis

Demonstrates arteriovenous malformations and berry aneurysms

Drawbacks

Complications occur in 2–25% of patients studied for cerebrovascular disease [4]; permanent neurological complications
occur in 0.5–3.0% depending on the center and the vessels
catheterized [7]

Contrast reactions and/or renal failure from contrast load rare

Death from myocardial infarction, arrhythmias, large hemi-
sphere infarcts occur in less than 0.5% [7]

Anticoagulation delayed by time required for arteriotomy to seal
(8–12 hours)

Comments

Availability of CT has obviated the need for angiography to document the presence of intracerebral hemorrhage

Risks of angiography should be weighed against potential benefit of therapies recommended on the basis of angiographic
findings

Multiple aneurysms may be demonstrated (not usual with CT)

Sensitivity

For major vessel thrombosis: *100%*; major vessel occlusions may
be embolic or thrombotic—distinction frequently depends on
clinical rather than angiographic features

For embolic disease: Studies within 48 hours of stroke show emboli in greater than *50%* of cases; later studies are often normal in embolic disease but persistently abnormal in thrombotic disease [5, 11]

For small vessel disease (lacunes or basilar branch disease): very low; embolus and small vessel thrombosis usually cannot be differentiated by angiography, which is often normal unless done sufficiently early to detect embolic material in small vessels

For intracranial aneurysms associated with subarachnoid hemorrhage: approximately 75–80%; 20% of arteriograms for subarachnoid hemorrhage show no clear vascular pathology—repeat angiography may lower this to 10–15%

For arteriovenous malformations: *100%*

Specificity

Angiography is the gold standard; specificity is very high by definition

Intravenous Digital Subtraction Angiography (IV DSA)

See discussion in Chapter 28, p. 145

Contribution of Magnetic Resonance Imaging [16, 20]

Detects the area of infarction much earlier than CT
Infarcted tissue and surrounding edema may have similar signal characteristics

References

1. Achar, V. S., Coe, R. P. K., and Marshall, J. Electroencephalography in the differential diagnosis of cerebral hemorrhage and infarction. *Lancet* 1:161, 1966.
2. Ackerman, R. H. Noninvasive carotid evaluation. *Stroke* 11:675, 1980.
3. Campbell, J. K., Houser, O. W., Stevens, J. C., et al. Computed tomography and radionuclide imaging in the evaluation of ischemic stroke. *Radiology* 126:695, 1978.
4. Faught, E., Trader, S. D., and Hanna, G. R. Cerebral complications of angiography for transient ischemia and stroke: Prediction of risk. *Neurology* 29:4, 1979.
5. Fieschi, C., and Bozzao, L. Transient embolic occlusion of the middle cerebral and internal carotid arteries in cerebral apoplexy. *J. Neurol. Neurosurg. Psychiatr.* 32:236, 1969.
6. Gado, M. H., Coleman, R. E., Merlis, A. L., et al. Comparison of computed tomography and radionuclide imaging in stroke. *Stroke* 7:109, 1976.
7. Hass, W. K., Fields, W. S., North, R. R., et al. Joint study of extracranial arterial occlusion. II. Arteriography techniques, sites and complications. *JAMA* 203:961, 1968.
8. James, E. M., Earnest, F., Forbes, G. S., et al. High-resolution dynamic ultrasound imaging of the carotid bifurcation: A prospective evaluation. *Radiology* 144:853, 1982.

9. Mills, C. M., Brant-Zawadzki, M., Crooks, L. E., et al. Nuclear magnetic resonance: Principles of blood flow imaging. *AJR* 142:165, 1984.

10. Modesti, L. M., and Binet, E. F. Value of computed tomography in the diagnosis and management of subarachnoid hemorrhage. *Neurosurgery* 3:151, 1978.

11. Mohr, J. P., Caplan, L. R., Melski, J. W., et al. The Harvard cooperative stroke registry: A prospective registry. *Neurology* 28:754, 1978.

12. Mohr, J. P., Kase, C. S., and Adams, R. D. Cerebrovascular Diseases. In R. G. Petersdorf, R. D. Adams, and E. Braunwald (Eds.). *Principles of Internal Medicine* (10th ed.). New York: McGraw-Hill, 1983. Pp. 2028–2060.

13. Mohr, J. P., and Kase, C. S. Cerebrovascular Disease. R. N. Rosenberg (Ed.). *The Clinical Neurosciences.* Vol. 1, Neurology. New York: Churchill Livingstone, 1983. Pp. 167–232.

14. O'Leary, D. H., Gibbons, G. W., and Pinel, D. F. Limitations of noninvasive testing in assessing the "occluded" carotid artery. *AJNR* 4:759, 1983.

15. O'Leary, D. H., Persson, A. V., and Clouse, M. E. Noninvasive testing for carotid artery stenosis. *A.J.N.R.* 2:437, 1981; *AJR* 137:1189, 1981.

16. Sipponen, J. T., Kaste, M., Ketonen, L., et al. Serial nuclear magnetic resonance (NMR) imaging in patients with cerebral infarction. *J. Comput. Assist. Tomogr.* 7:585, 1983.

17. Weisberg, L. A. Computed tomographic enhancement patterns in cerebral infarction. *Arch. Neurol.* 37:21, 1980.

18. Wirth, F. P. Computerized tomography and subarachnoid hemorrhage. *JAMA* 241:563, 1979.

19. Wolverson, M. K., Heiberg, E., Sundaram, E., et al. Carotid atherosclerosis: High resolution real-time sonography correlated with angiography. *AJR* 140:355, 1983.

20. Zabramski, J. M., Spetzler, R. F., and Kaufman, B. Magnetic resonance imaging: Comparative study of radiofrequency pulse techniques in the evaluation of focal cerebral ischemia. *Neurosurgery* 16:502, 1985.

30

Headache

Amir A. Zamani

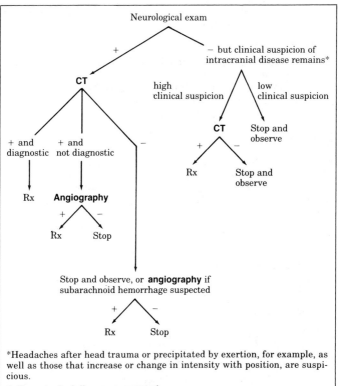

Neurological exam

+ / − but clinical suspicion of
intracranial disease remains*

CT

high clinical suspicion / low clinical suspicion

+ and diagnostic / + and not diagnostic / −

CT / Stop and observe

+ / −

Rx / Stop and observe

Rx / **Angiography**

+ / −

Rx / Stop

Stop and observe, or **angiography** if subarachnoid hemorrhage suspected

+ / −

Rx / Stop

*Headaches after head trauma or precipitated by exertion, for example, as well as those that increase or change in intensity with position, are suspicious.

A. Neurological disease suspected

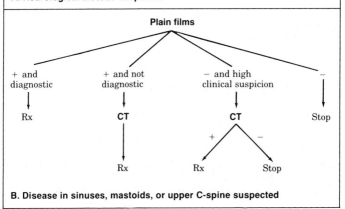

Plain films

+ and diagnostic / + and not diagnostic / − and high clinical suspicion / −

Rx / **CT** / **CT** / Stop

Rx / + / −

Rx / Stop

B. Disease in sinuses, mastoids, or upper C-spine suspected

Individual experiencing
> Pain or discomfort from pain-sensitive structures inside cranial cavity
>
> Pain referred to the head from adjacent structures with or without neurological findings

Typical Disorder(s)

Extracranial: migraines; headaches due to tension or to diseases of the paranasal sinuses

Intracranial: traumatic, neoplastic, inflammatory

General: arterial hypertension

Plain Films

Useful primarily for detecting trauma, bone destruction, or calcified lesions within the brain

Frequently useful in diagnosing meningiomas because of vascular marking in cranial vault or because of localized hyperostosis

Useful for diagnosing sinusitis, except in area of sphenoid sinus

Drawbacks

Low diagnostic yield

Generally unrewarding unless intracranial disease produces calcification or is the product of skull trauma

Sensitivity

For nontraumatic headaches: very low yield (less than 5%), even in patients with positive neurological findings [6]

False negatives can occur
> In nearly all intracranial processes that do not produce calcification or alter bony structures

Specificity

Except for diseases of paranasal sinuses: quite nonspecific

False positives can occur
> If a cranial lesion is interpreted as a brain lesion

Head Computed Tomography (CT)

Examination of choice for headaches associated with some neurological signs, overall yield about *30%* [9, 14]

Examination of choice if headache believed to be a consequence of trauma

Detects intracranial disease such as neoplasm, infarction, or hemorrhage [1, 21]

Establishes the presence of more than a single lesion

Precisely demonstrates shift in the midline and other anatomical abnormalities

Better for detecting supratentorial lesions rather than those in the posterior cranial fossa

Drawbacks

Low yield (essentially 0%) with headaches unassociated with neurological signs or symptoms [9, 14]

Potential contrast reactions (total 5%) [19]

Sensitivity

For detecting intracranial masses in general and tumors in particular: 95–98% [5]

For detecting subarachnoid hemorrhage: variable, depending on the number of red blood cells in spinal fluid; may be 95–100% initially [2, 20], dropping to 85% by 5 days and to 50% after 1 week [20]

For detecting chronic subdural hematomas: somewhat less than for acute processes, 97% [1]

False negatives can occur

With lesions having the same attenuation value as surrounding normal brain

With small lesions adjacent to the bony calvarium

Specificity

For showing normal intracranial structures or benign disease in patients suspected of malignant tumor, using contrast-enhanced scans: 97% [5]

For showing normal intracranial structures or benign disease in patients suspected of malignant tumor, using noncontrast scans: 93% [5]

For showing normal intracranial structures in patients suspected of chronic subdural disease in general: greater than 96%

False positive readings for specific diagnoses can occur

If infarct is mistaken for tumor (or vice versa)

With old scanners if cysts or tumors are mistaken for subdural hematomas [11]

Cerebral Angiography

Definitively diagnoses vascular lesions

Clarifies the blood supply to neoplasms and indicates their distribution and localization

Helpful in surgery by providing a vascular map

Initially considered more sensitive in comparison to noncontrast CT studies, but these data are becoming controversial; about the same sensitivity as contrast studies [5]

May define small lesions not resolvable by CT

Drawbacks

Invasive, with total complication rate of 1.4% (hematomas, transient neurological deficits) and permanent and major CNS complications or death of 0.06% [16]

Sensitivity

For detecting intracranial masses, tumors in particular: *96%* [5]
For detecting aneurysms associated with subarachnoid hemorrhage: *95%*
False negatives can occur in brain tumor detection
    Depending on location (e.g., parasagittal tumors are difficult to detect)
    In very small lesions
    In the presence of multiple lesions: Examination may detect only the largest
False negatives can occur in aneurysm detection
    Usually because of an incomplete examination

Specificity

Angiography is the gold standard: Specificity is very high by definition

Radionuclide (RN) Brain Scan

With dynamic scanning can assess flow in major arteries
Useful for early subdural hematomas if CT attenuation value of hematoma approximates that of normal brain
Useful for vascular lesions, particularly meningiomas

Drawbacks

Three-hour delay between injection and imaging
Very poor resolution compared to CT
Poor ability to differentiate benign from malignant processes
Poor sensitivity for acute subdural processes: Dynamic studies have variable accuracy in acute phase and static studies do not become abnormal for at least 5 days after event, best after 10

Comment

This study is not included explicitly in the algorithm because of the general availability and reliability of CT; however, those institutions not having CT can benefit from radionuclide imaging

Sensitivity

For detecting intracranial masses: *80–85%* [3]
For detecting chronic subdural hematomas: greater than *85–90%* [8, 10], unilateral more accurately than bilateral

False negatives can occur

For mass lesions because of location, particularly perisellar and posterior fossa lesions

For subdural hematomas because of early age or bilaterality

For any lesion of small size

Specificity

For showing normal intracranial structures in patients suspected of mass lesion: lower than that of CT

For showing normal intracranial structures in patients suspected of aneurysmal bleed or subdural hematoma: lower than that of CT

Contribution of Magnetic Resonance Imaging [7, 15]

Provides fine anatomical detail for brain imaging

Posterior fossa and brain stem lesions in particular are well shown

May soon become the primary modality for imaging intracranial pathology

References

1. Abrams, H. L., and McNeil, B. J. Medical implications of computed tomography ("CAT scanning"). *N. Engl. J. Med.* 298:255; 310, 1978.

2. Adams, H. P., Jr., Kassell, N. F., Torner, J. C., et al. CT and clinical correlations in recent aneurysmal subarachnoid hemorrhage: A preliminary report of the cooperative aneurysm study. *Neurology* 33:981, 1983.

3. Alderson, P. O., Gado, M. H., and Siegel, B. A. Computerized cranial tomography and radionuclide imaging in the detection of intracranial mass lesions. *Semin. Nucl. Med.* 7:161, 1977.

4. Anderson, R. E., and Millikan, C. H. Headache. In R. L. Eisenberg and J. R. Amberg (Eds.). *Critical Diagnostic Pathways in Radiology: An Algorithm Approach* (1st ed.). Philadelphia: Lippincott, 1981. Pp. 312–319.

5. Baker, H. L., Jr., Houser, O. W., and Campbell, J. K. National Cancer Institute study: Evaluation of computed tomography in the diagnosis of intracranial neoplasms. 1. Overall results. *Radiology* 136:91, 1980.

6. Bessen, H. A., and Rothstein, R. J. Futility of skull radiography for nontraumatic conditions. *Ann. Emerg. Med.* 11:605, 1982.

7. Brant-Zawadzki, M., Davis, P. L., Crooks, L. E., et al. NMR demonstration of cerebral abnormalities: Comparison with CT. *AJNR* 4:117, 1983.

8. Brown, R., Weber, P. M., and dos Remedios, L. V. Dynamic/static brain scintigraphy: An effective screening test for subdural hematoma. *Radiology* 117:355, 1975.
9. Carrera, G. F., Gerson, D. E., Schnur, J., et al. Computed tomography of the brain in patients with headache or temporal lobe epilepsy: Findings and cost-effectiveness. *J. Comput. Assist. Tomogr.* 1:200, 1977.
10. Cowan, R. J., and Maynard, C. D. Trauma to the brain and extracranial structures. *Semin. Nucl. Med.* 4:319, 1974.
11. Forbes, G. S., Sheedy, P. F., II, Piepgras, D. G., et al. Computed tomography in the evaluation of subdural hematomas. *Radiology* 126:143, 1978.
12. Kandalaft, N., Diehl, J., and Neuwelt, E. A. Nonneoplastic intracranial lesions simulating neoplasms on computed tomographic scan: Excellent sensitivity with limited specificity. *JAMA* 248:2166, 1982.
13. Knaus, W. A., Wagner, D. P., and Davis, D. O. CT for headache: Cost/benefit for subarachnoid hemorrhage. *AJR* 136:537, 1981.
14. Larson, E. B., Omenn, G. S., and Lewis, H. Diagnostic evaluation of headache: Impact of computerized tomography and cost-effectiveness. *JAMA* 243:359, 1980.
15. Lee, B. C. P., Kneeland, J. B., Deck, M. D. F., et al. Posterior fossa lesions: Magnetic resonance imaging. *Radiology* 153:137, 1984.
16. Mani, R. L., Eisenberg, R. L., McDonald, E. J., Jr., et al. Complications of catheter cerebral arteriography: Analysis of 5,000 procedures. 1. Criteria and incidence. *AJR* 131:861, 1978.
17. Plum, F. Headache. In J. B. Wyngaarden and L. H. Smith (Eds.). *Cecil Textbook of Medicine* (16th ed.). Philadelphia: Saunders, 1982. Pp. 1948–1953.
18. Sargent, J. D., Lawson, R. C., Solbach, P., et al. Use of CT scans in an out-patient headache population: An evaluation. *Headache* 19:388, 1979.
19. Shehadi, W. H. Contrast media adverse reactions: Occurrence, recurrence and distribution patterns. *Radiology* 143:11, 1982.
20. van Gijn, J., and van Dongen, K. J. The time course of aneurysmal hemorrhage on computed tomograms. *Neuroradiology* 23:153, 1982.
21. Weisberg, L. A. Computed tomography in the diagnosis of intracranial disease. *Ann. Intern. Med.* 91:87, 1979.

31

Seizures

Hani A. A. F. Haykal

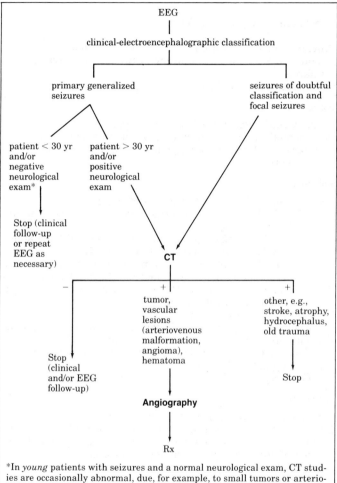

*In *young* patients with seizures and a normal neurological exam, CT studies are occasionally abnormal, due, for example, to small tumors or arteriovenous malformations

Typical Patient

Individual experiencing convulsive disorders characterized by abrupt transient motor, sensory, psychic, or autonomic symptoms

Typical Disorder(s)

Focal brain disorders
Mass lesions

Computed Tomography (CT)

Provides superb resolution of intracranial anatomy
Provides high diagnostic accuracy in tumors, hemorrhage, and infarcts
Diminishes the need for invasive examinations

Drawbacks

In idiopathic epilepsy, CT is usually negative
Rare complications, occasional contrast reactions, and/or secondary renal failure occur, but serious reactions only 1 in 14,000 [4]

Sensitivity

For patients with electrochemical forms of epilepsy [7]:
  10% of patients with idiopathic epilepsy will have abnormal CTs [8–9]
  61% with secondary generalized epilepsy will have abnormal CTs (in most cases atrophy [2, 13, 15])
  30% [1, 15] to *60%* [6, 8, 9] of patients with partial generalized epilepsy will have abnormal CTs, and most of these will have focal lesions; the incidence of abnormal CT findings increases with age [15]
For post-traumatic epilepsy:
  About *85%* of patients will show focal or diffuse CT lesion
For patients with seizures, secondary to tumor:
  Sensitivity is extremely high (100% in one series [8]), averaging *95–98%* [1]
  False negatives for tumors occur rarely

Specificity

For individuals under age 30: virtually *100%*
Especially for those over age 60 the specificity is lower because many have global atrophy; some have focal atrophy in the absence of any abnormality leading to seizures
False positives for tumors can occur
  If chronic hemorrhage is mistaken for tumor

Angiography

Depicts vascular morphology with great precision
Demonstrates not only mass lesions and aneurysms but discrete occlusions of vessels
Frequently permits a definitive diagnosis
May be essential for management and treatment planning

Drawbacks

Mass lesions are shown by displacement of vessels rather than directly

Total complication rate, 1.4% (hematomas, transient neurological deficits); permanent and major CNS complications or death, 0.06% [12]

Sensitivity

For diagnosis of vascular lesions (AVM, hemangioma): very high
For diagnosis of chronic subdural hematomas: high

Specificity

For differentiating vascular lesions and subdural hematomas from normal: nearly *100%*

Contribution of Magnetic Resonance Imaging [3, 16]

May demonstrate lesions such as gliosis or tumors not always recognized on CT

Delineates vascular malformations without contrast injection

References

1. Baker, H. L., Houser, W., and Campbell, J. K. NCI study: Evaluation of CT in the diagnosis of intracranial neoplasms. *Radiology* 136:91, 1980.
2. Bogdanoff, B. M., Stafford, C. R., Green, L., et al. Computerized transaxial tomography in the evaluation of patients with focal epilepsy. *Neurology* 25:1013, 1975.
3. Brant-Zawadzki, M., Badami, J. P., Mills, C. M., et al. Primary intracranial tumor imaging: A comparison of magnetic resonance and CT. *Radiology* 150:435, 1984.
4. Broderick, T. W. Contrast Material Reactions. In G. W. Friedland, R. Filly, and M. L. Goris (Eds.). *Uroradiology*. New York: Churchill Livingstone, 1983.
5. Earnest, F., IV, Forbes, G., Sandok, B. A., et al. Complications of cerebral angiography: Prospective assessment of risk. *AJR* 142:247, 1984.
6. Gall, M. V., Becker, H., and Hacker, H. Summary: Computerized transverse axial tomography in epilepsy. No. 3. *Epilepsia* 17:339, 1976.
7. Gastaut, H. Clinical and electroencephalographical classification of epileptic seizures. *Epilepsia* 11:102, 1970.
8. Gastaut, H., and Gastaut, J.-L. Computerized transverse axial tomography in epilepsy. *Epilepsia* 17:325, 1976.
9. Gastaut, H., and Gastaut, J.-L. Computerized Axial Tomography in Epilepsy. In J. K. Penry (Ed.). *Epilepsy: The Ninth International Symposium*. New York: Raven, 1977. Pp. 5–15.
10. Hounsfield, G. N. Computerized transverse axial scanning (tomography). Part I. Description of system. *Br. J. Radiol.* 46:1016, 1973.

11. Krupp, M. A., and Chatton, M. J. (Eds.). *Current Medical Diagnosis and Treatment.* Los Altos, Cal.: Lange Medical Publications, 1981. Pp. 570–575.
12. Mani, R. L., Eisenberg, R. L., McDonald, E. J., Jr., et al. Complications of catheter cerebral arteriography: Analysis of 5,000 procedures. 1. Criteria and incidence. *AJR* 131:881, 1978.
13. McGahan, J. P., Dublin, A. B., and Hill, R. P. The evaluation of seizure disorders by computerized tomography. *J. Neurosurg.* 50:328, 1979.
14. Penry, J. K., and Porter, R. J. Epilepsy: Mechanisms and therapy. *Med. Clin. North Am.* 63:801, 1979.
15. Scollo-Lavizzari, G., and Balmer, C. Electroencephalography and computerized transaxial tomography in patients with temporal lobe epilepsy. *Eur. Neurol.* 19:33, 1980.
16. Sostman, H. D., Spencer, D. D., Gore, J. C., et al. Preliminary observations on magnetic resonance imaging in refractory epilepsy. *Magnetic Resonance Imaging* 2:301, 1984.

Head Trauma, Including Cervical Spine Injury

Michael L. Lewis

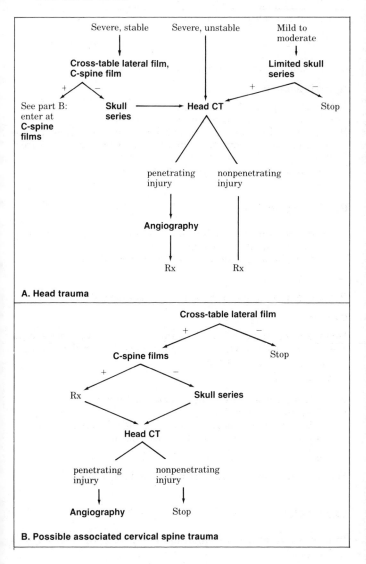

A. Head trauma

B. Possible associated cervical spine trauma

Typical Patient

Individual experiencing mild to moderate or severe head trauma, with possible incidental injury to the cervical spine;

163

severe head trauma includes:
  A history of unconsciousness, retrograde amnesia; the use
    of anticoagulants
  Clinical suspicion of skull penetration
  Focal neurological symptoms
  Bony malalignment or bulging
  Discharge from ear or nose, discoloration of ear, bilateral
    black eyes
  Stupor or coma, irregular breathing

Typical Disorder(s)

Soft tissue injury to scalp or face
Skull fractures and intracranial injury or bleeding
Intracranial abnormalities: cerebral contusion, subdural hema-
  toma, epidural hematoma, subarachnoid hemorrhage, direct
  injury to brain substance
For cervical spine: fractures and dislocations

Cervical Spine Films

Lateral film is useful for initial evaluation (i.e., bone integrity,
  spinal alignment, soft tissue swelling) [3]
Indicated whenever brain trauma is suspected

Drawbacks

Reveals only trauma to the spine, not the cord itself

Comments

Head trauma and cervical spine injury are highly associated [3]
The patient with cervical spine injury must be handled carefully
  during this examination

Sensitivity

For detecting fractures and dislocations: high
False negatives can occur
  When there are hairline fractures with displacements
  If C7 or T1 is not adequately visualized

Specificity

For showing normal structures: approaching *100%*

Skull Series

Indicates site of fracture and, most importantly, whether it is
  depressed

Drawbacks

Cannot detect intracerebral pathology

Yield is relatively low in the absence of symptoms from skull trauma [4, 5]

Comments

Site of fracture may be important in determining discharge vs. in-hospital observation and possible CT scan in asymptomatic patients (i.e., location adjacent to large venous sinus or middle meningeal artery increases risk)

Even if a skull fracture is demonstrated, the important question concerns trauma to the underlying brain

The use of skull radiography in head trauma is somewhat controversial. The 1979 edition of *Cecil Textbook of Medicine* states that "roentgenographic examination of the skull should be performed without undue delay in all cases of injury to the head." The 1982 edition of the same book does not even mention skull radiography.

Radionuclide brain scanning is sometimes used for patients suffering the sequelae of head trauma (see Chap. 30, p. 156) but is not the modality of choice for acute disease

Sensitivity

For fractures: high

For brain damage: low

Specificity

For showing normal bone: high

Head Computed Tomography (CT)

Detects bony abnormalities

Detects intracranial hemorrhage

Reveals the anatomy and position of the ventricular system and associated brain tissue

Demonstrates collections of blood and their effect on the brain

May detect unsuspected pre-existing condition that contributed to trauma (e.g., brain tumor leading to seizure, chronic cysts, old subdural hematomas)

Drawbacks

Low yield without clinical indication of brain trauma

Rare complications; occasional contrast reactions and/or secondary renal failure occur, with serious reactions only 1 in 14,000 [7]

May miss a fracture parallel to plane of beam or in area not specifically studied

Comment

Cranial computed tomography has replaced radionuclide scintigraphy because its sensitivity and specificity are better; occasionally, however, an isodense chronic subdural hematoma
may be missed on CT and detected on RN scan

Sensitivity

For detecting acute subdural hematomas: high
For detecting chronic subdural hematomas: 97% [1]
For detecting subarachnoid hemorrhage: variable, but higher
with large numbers of red blood cells in spinal fluid; may be
as high as 95–100% initially [2, 12], dropping off to 85% by 5
days and to 50% by 1 week [12]
For detecting epidural bleed: high
For detecting depressed skull fractures: very high
False negatives for all diseases can occur
With motion artifacts

Specificity

For showing normal intracranial structures for patients suspected of acute subdural hematoma, chronic subdural hematoma, epidural or subarachnoid bleed, or depressed skull fracture: high [8]
False positives can occur
With motion artifacts

Angiography

Precisely depicts the vascular anatomy of the brain
Clearly defines vascular injury from a penetrating wound
Delineates intracerebral hemorrhage and its effect on the ven-
tricular system, but not as well as CT with contrast enhance-
ment
Precisely diagnoses the nature and extent of vascular disease
and anomalies
Provides a vascular map for the surgeon

Drawbacks

Total complication rate, 1.4% (hematomas, transient neurological deficits; permanent and major CNS complications or
death, 0.06% [10]

Sensitivity

For detecting subdural hematomas: high [6]
For detecting intracerebral hematomas, high but CT more precise

Specificity

Is generally considered the gold standard: specificity high [6]
False positives can occur
    When brain atrophy simulates subdural hematoma

Contribution of Magnetic Resonance Imaging [9]

Clearly demonstrates cerebral edema and may also show subtle
    changes in white matter after trauma, which are not always
    detected by CT
Demonstrates intra- or extracerebral hematoma

References

1. Abrams, H. L., and McNeil, B. J. Medical implications of computed tomography ("CAT scanning"). *N. Engl. J. Med.* 298:255, 1978.
2. Adams, H. P., Jr., Kassell, N. F., Torner, J. C., et al. CT and clinical correlations in recent aneurysmal subarachnoid hemorrhage: A preliminary report of the Cooperative Aneurysm Study. *Neurology* 33:981, 1983.
3. Alker, G. J., Jr., Oh, Y. S., and Leslie, E. V. High cervical spine and craniocervical junction injuries in fatal traffic accidents: A radiologic study. *Orthop. Clin. North Am.* 9;1003, 1978.
4. Balasubramaniam, S., Kapadia, T., Campbell, J. A., et al. Efficacy of skull radiography. *Am. J. Surg.* 142:366, 1981.
5. Bell, R. S., and Loop, J. W. The utility and futility of radiographic skull examination for trauma. *N. Engl. J. Med.* 284:236, 1971.
6. Ben-Menachem, Y. *Angiography in Trauma: A Work Atlas.* Philadelphia: Saunders, 1981.
7. Broderick, T. W. Contrast Material Reactions. In G. W. Friedland, R. Filly, and M. L. Goris (Eds.). *Uroradiology.* New York: Churchill Livingstone, 1983.
8. Forbes, G. S., Sheedy, P. F., II, Piepgras, D. G., et al. Computed tomography in the evaluation of subdural hematomas. *Radiology* 126:143, 1978.
9. Han, J. S., Kaufman, B., Alfidi, R. J., et al. Head trauma evaluated by magnetic resonance and computed tomography: A comparison. *Radiology* 150:71, 1984.
10. Mani, R. L., Eisenberg, R. L., McDonald, E. J., Jr., et al. Complications of catheter cerebral arteriography: Analysis of 5,000 procedures. 1. Criteria and incidence. *AJR* 131:881, 1978.
11. Shehadi, W. H. Contrast media adverse reactions: Occurrence, recurrence and distribution patterns. *Radiology* 143:11, 1982.
12. van Gijn, J., and van Dongen, K. J. The time course of aneurysmal hemorrhage on computed tomography. *Neuroradiology* 23:153, 1982.

Low Back Pain

Ay-Ming Wang

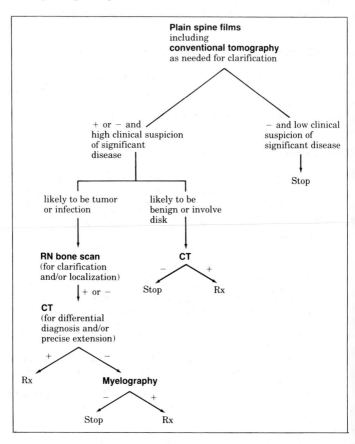

Typical Patient

Individual experiencing persistent low back pain that is local, referred, radicular, or arising secondarily (protective muscular spasm); the pain may be acute, intermittent, or chronic

Typical Disorder(s)

Disk herniation and degenerative disk disease
Spinal stenosis
Spondylosis, spondylolisthesis, spondylolysis
Infections or tumors
Trauma: fracture, epidural hematoma

Post-laminectomy scarring, adhesive arachnoiditis
Uncommon disorders

Comments

95% of patients with low back pain syndrome have temporary symptoms for which no radiological examinations are necessary

In one study [10] disk herniation accounted for more than 50% of pathological findings; all other causes occurred less than 10% of the time

Clinical diagnoses are accurate less than 50% of the time

Plain Films

Excellent demonstration of gross anatomy [4]
May define the cause of low back pain
Identifies areas of disk narrowing and zygapophyseal joint changes
Clarifies the presence of infection and/or neoplasm
Inexpensive, rapidly obtained, easily interpreted

Drawbacks

Cannot define intraspinal canal soft tissue lesions
Cannot identify early bone destruction
Frequently inadequate for definitive diagnosis
Significant radiation dose to critical organs

Comment

Conventional films are the essential first step in diagnostic work-up for all patients with persistent low back pain

Sensitivity

Exact figures difficult to obtain, but probably about *60–70%*
False negatives can occur
    Due to the scarcity of direct plain film findings

Specificity

Very high

Conventional Tomography

Permits precise visualization of fine details of osseous structures
May confirm findings visible but of uncertain significance on conventional films

Drawbacks

Limited detail of soft tissue structure
Fails to provide cross-sectional studies

Sensitivity

No specific data available but
> High for trauma with fractures and for spondylosis, spondylolisthesis, and spondylolysis
>
> Moderate for tumor or infection
>
> Low (or sometimes zero) for disk herniation, epidural hematoma

Specificity

No specific data available but if specific signs are used as criterion for abnormality (e.g., lytic destruction), high

Lumbar Spine Computed Tomography (CT)

Excellent demonstration of cross-sectional anatomy

Defines both bony and soft tissue components

Detects bone destruction at an earlier stage than conventional tomography

Demonstrates normal lumbar disks, bulging anuli, herniated nuclei pulposus

Particularly good for diskitis, spondylosis, and spinal stenosis

As effective as myelography for most lumbar diseases

Drawbacks

Not useful for diagnosing epidural fibrosis

Interpretations sometimes difficult in postoperative patients

Patient cooperation required for 10 seconds per slice

May require contrast agent (e.g., low-dose metrizamide intrathecal injection or intravenous contrast enhancement)

Transient side effects can occur with metrizamide-enhanced CT: headaches, 31–68%; nausea and vomiting, 9–38% [1]

Comments

High-resolution CT scan is preferable, if available

Sensitivity

For disk herniations: *97%* (29 of 30 patients) [5]

For spinal stenosis and spondylosis: approaching *100%*

False negatives can occur
> From failing to distinguish spondylosis and bulging anulus from herniated nucleus pulposus

Specificity

Generally high, but 32% of patients with suspected herniated disks had false positive readings [5]

False positives can occur
> From failing to distinguish spondylosis and bulging anulus from herniated nucleus pulposus

Radionuclide (RN) Bone Scan

Detects alterations in bone relatively early compared to plain films [9]

Provides examination of nearly the entire skeleton and, if positive, indicates appropriate CT level

Useful in follow up to detect bone activity after therapy

Drawbacks

Relatively poor resolution compared with computed tomography

Relatively low yield in most settings with low back pain, particularly those caused by herniated disk and degenerative disk disease

Cannot be used for intraspinal processes

Sensitivity

For metastatic disease: extremely high, probably highest of all radiographical modalities

For osteomyelitis: very high, especially when coupled with gallium scan (see Chap. 43, p. 215)

Specificity

Low: nearly all benign processes (arthritis, for example) will give positive bone scans

Metrizamide Myelography

Detects intrathecal space-occupying lesions and extradural compression

Gives good description of subarachnoid space

Localizes level of cord compression precisely

Drawbacks

Contraindicated for patients with bleeding tendency and allergy to contrast material

Complications (headache, nausea, vomiting) nearly half the time [6]; seizure, anaphylactic reaction, and epidural hemorrhage can occasionally occur

Less useful than CT for diagnosing diskitis

Sensitivity

For herniated disks: *93%* (28 of 30 patients) [5]

For spinal stenosis: approaching *100%*

For spondylolysis: high

False negatives can occur

> From failing to distinguish spondylosis and bulging anulus from herniated nucleus pulposus

Specificity

For patients subsequently shown to have herniated disk: *64%* (9 of 25 false positive readings) [5]
False positives can occur
> From failing to distinguish spondylosis and bulging anulus from herniated nucleus pulposus

Contribution of Magnetic Resonance Imaging [3, 8]

Competes with CT in defining normal and abnormal invertebral disks and spinal anatomy

References

1. Baker, R. A., Hillman, B. J., McLennan, J. E., et al. Sequelae of metrizamide myelography in 200 examinations. *AJR* 130:499, 1978.
2. Cailliet, R. *Low Back Pain Syndrome* (3rd ed.). Philadelphia: Davis, 1981.
3. Chafetz, N. I., Genant, H. K., Moon, K. L., et al. Recognition of lumbar disk herniation with NMR. *AJR* 141:1153, 1983.
4. Epstein, B. S. *The Spine. A Radiological Text and Atlas* (4th ed.). Philadelphia: Lea & Febiger, 1976.
5. Haughton, V. M., Eldevik, O. P., Magnaes, B., et al. A prospective comparison of computed tomography and myelography in the diagnosis of herniated lumbar disks. *Radiology* 142:103, 1982.
6. Kieffer, S. A., Binet, E. F., Esquerra, J. V., et al. Contrast agents for myelography: Clinical and radiological evaluation of Amipaque and Pantopaque. *Radiology* 129:695, 1978.
7. Livermore, N. B., III. Low Back Pain Syndrome: A Clinical Overview. In H. K. Genant, N. Chafetz, and C. A. Helms (Eds.). *Computed Tomography of the Lumbar Spine*. Berkeley: University of California, 1982. Pp. 1–14.
8. Modic, M. T., Pavlicek, W., Weinstein, M. A., et al. Magnetic resonance imaging of intervertebral disk disease. *Radiology* 152:103, 1984.
9. Schütte, H. E., and Park, W. M. The diagnostic value of bone scintigraphy in patients with low back pain. *Skeletal Radiol.* 10:1, 1983.
10. Van Damme, W., Hessels, G., Verhelst, M., et al. Relative efficacy of clinical examination, electromyography, plain film radiography, myelography and lumbar phlebography in the diagnosis of low back pain and sciatica. *Neuroradiology* 18:109, 1979.

Acute Spine Trauma

Hani A. A. F. Haykal

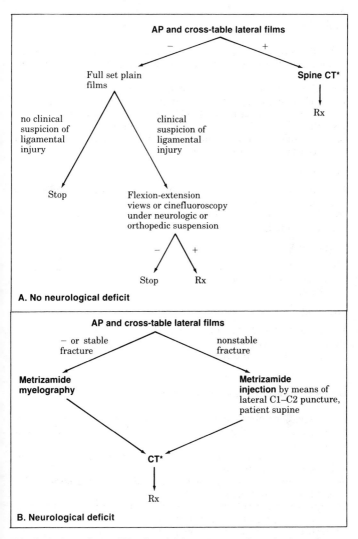

A. No neurological deficit

AP and cross-table lateral films

− / +

Full set plain films / Spine CT*

Spine CT* → Rx

no clinical suspicion of ligamental injury → Stop

clinical suspicion of ligamental injury → Flexion-extension views or cinefluoroscopy under neurologic or orthopedic suspension

− Stop / + Rx

B. Neurological deficit

AP and cross-table lateral films

− or stable fracture → **Metrizamide myelography**

nonstable fracture → **Metrizamide injection** by means of lateral C1–C2 puncture, patient supine

CT* → Rx

*Ideally, high-resolution CT with multiplanar image reformation is used

Typical Patient

Individual with a possible fracture of the spine, ranging from the cervical spine to the lumbar spine

Typical Disorder(s)

Flexion, extension, axial compression or rotational injuries

Plain Films

Initially, only anteroposterior and cross-table lateral views are
   obtained to protect cord from trauma due to excessive manipulation
Useful for screening for disease site before CT
In cervical spine, useful for recognizing malalignment, particularly if only the transverse CT sections are available
Excellent for transverse fractures of odontoid
May provide adequate information to preclude other studies,
   particularly if completely negative

Drawbacks

Good quality radiographs are sometimes technically difficult to
   obtain on immobilized patients
Precise relationship of fracture to spinal canal is not always
   fully defined

Sensitivity

High, but poorer than that of CT: missed 5 of 15 fractures [2]
False negatives can occur
   From patient motion

Specificity

High, but lower than that of CT [5]
False positives can occur
   From patient motion

Spine Computed Tomography (CT)

Visualizes vertebral bodies and posterior elements in axial
   plane, and by reformatting, in sagittal, coronal, and oblique
   planes [3]
Defines degree and location of fragmentation at fracture site
   better than plain films
Assesses spinal column status, including hemorrhage within
   canal and disk herniation [4, 5]
Permits diagnosis of injury to associated organs (intrathoracic,
   intrapelvic) and in paraspinal soft tissue area
Metrizamide-enhanced CT permits diagnosis of spinal cord injury including swelling, maceration, and hemorrhage, although the use in unstable fractures is questionable

Drawbacks

In absence of reformatting in many planes, availability of axial images alone makes interpretation of subtle alignment difficult [3]

Transient side effects (headaches, nausea, and vomiting) can occur with metrizamide-enhanced CT [1]

Comments

To maintain proper traction, traumatized patient should be transferred under supervision of a neurosurgeon or orthopedist

To reduce motion artifacts, which may significantly degrade image, patient should be given an analgesic (when not contraindicated)

High-resolution CT with multiplanar image reformation is preferable, but not available everywhere

Examination is best reserved for detailed study of limited spinal segment, especially when thin slices are used

Sensitivity

Considerably higher than conventional films: In 5 out of 15 patients with spine trauma CT showed fractures not seen on plain films, and for 9 of the 15, abnormalities of the spinal canal were found [2]

False negatives can occur

In regions adjacent to dense bone (e.g., beyond pedicle) due to partial volume effect

Specificity

High: Can verify that questionable lesions on plain films are normal

False positives can occur due to

Patient motion

Metallic traction devices

Metrizamide Myelography

Gives excellent depiction of subarachnoid space
Defines extradural and intradural abnormalities clearly
Localizes the level of cord compression precisely

Drawbacks

Does not depict the relationship of osseous fragment to cord as well as does CT

Possibility of cord trauma resulting from excessive manipulation in the setting of an unstable spine

Possibility of side effects: postexamination headache, 62%; nausea and/or vomiting associated with metrizamide, 38% [1]

Sensitivity

For defining cause and localizing level of cord compression: approaching *100%*

Specificity

Low specificity for cause of cord compression
False positives can occur
> From faulty myelographic technique; injection of contrast into subdural or epidural space instead of subarachnoid space will give the appearance of tumor or cord compression

References

1. Baker, R. A., Hillman, B. J., McLennan, J. E., et al. Sequelae of metrizamide myelography in 200 examinations. *AJR* 130:499, 1978.
2. Brant-Zawadski, M., Miller, E. M., and Federle, M. P. CT in the evaluation of spine trauma. *AJR* 136:369, 1981.
3. Cacayorin, E. D., and Kieffer, S. A. Applications and limitations of computed tomography of the spine. *Radiol. Clin. North Am.* 20:185, 1982.
4. Donovan Post, M. J., Green, B. A., Quencer, R. M., et al. The value of computed tomography in spinal trauma. *Spine* 7:417, 1982.
5. Newton, T. H., and Potts, D. G. (Eds.). *Computed Tomography of the Spine and Spinal Cord.* San Anselmo, Cal.: Clavadel Press, 1983. Pp. 186–206.

Spinal Cord Compression

Calvin L. Rumbaugh

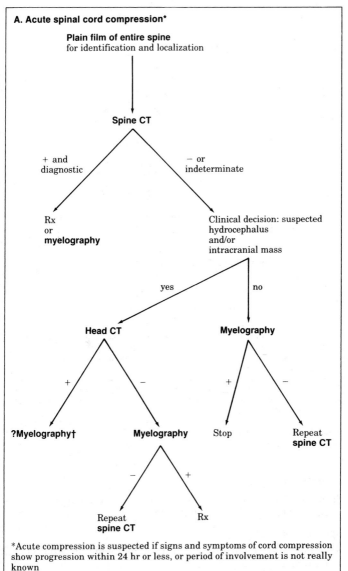

A. Acute spinal cord compression*

Plain film of entire spine
for identification and localization

↓

Spine CT

+ and
diagnostic

− or
indeterminate

Rx
or
myelography

Clinical decision: suspected
hydrocephalus
and/or
intracranial mass

yes

no

Head CT

Myelography

+

−

+

−

?Myelography†

Myelography

Stop

Repeat
spine CT

−

+

Repeat
spine CT

Rx

*Acute compression is suspected if signs and symptoms of cord compression
show progression within 24 hr or less, or period of involvement is not really
known
†If head CT is positive for hydrocephalus or intracranial mass, the need for
myelography should be re-evaluated with neurosurgical consultation

177

B. Chronic spinal cord compression

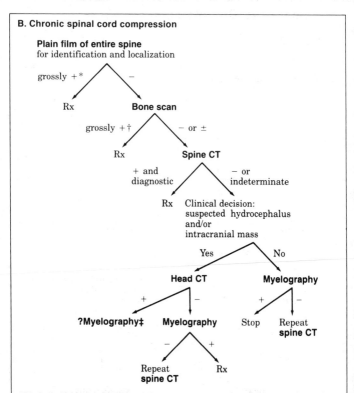

Plain film of entire spine
for identification and localization

grossly + *

Rx   **Bone scan**

grossly + †   − or ±

Rx   **Spine CT**

+ and
diagnostic   − or
indeterminate

Rx Clinical decision:
suspected hydrocephalus
and/or
intracranial mass

Yes   No

Head CT   **Myelography**

+ −   + −

?Myelography‡ **Myelography**   Stop Repeat
spine CT

− +

Repeat   Rx
spine CT

*If plain film exam shows such extensive bone destruction and soft tissue changes that complete spinal canal obstruction seems highly probable, and if site is compatible with symptoms and signs, the radiological evaluation is complete at this point

†If bone scan is not only positive for clinical area of suspected cord compression but also shows multiple lesions characteristic of metastatic disease (and no evidence of septicemia), the radiological exam should be discontinued if no additional information is required

‡If head CT is positive for hydrocephalus or intracranial mass, the need for myelography should be re-evaluated with neurosurgical consultation

Typical Patient

Individual experiencing pain, weakness, autonomic dysfunction, or sensory loss, including ataxia

Typical Disorder(s)

Primary or secondary tumor in bone or in epidural space (e.g., lymphoma)
Trauma
Inflammatory process
Degenerative spine disease

Comments

Even if symptoms appear localized, multiple lesions may exist (some without symptoms); therefore plain film surveys of the thoracic and cervical spine are desirable (and so may be myelography)

Intracranial lesions may mimic symptoms of cord compression

Plain Films

Important screening procedure for all cases

Permits identification of presence and location of disease in some cases

Drawbacks

Not sensitive

About 50% of cortical bone must be destroyed before disease appears on film

Sensitivity

For primary or secondary tumor: low [4]

For inflammatory disease: low [2]

For degenerative disease: high [6, 13]

For trauma: high [3]

False negatives can occur

    For tumors that do not show bone changes

    For early infectious processes

Specificity

In general, high; but cannot always differentiate infection from tumor [2]

Bone Scan

Very good for surveying entire vertebral skeleton for site and presence of disease

Can serve as guide for CT studies

Drawbacks

Low specificity, particularly in bones with coexistent or previous disease

Poor resolution

2- to 3-hour delay between injection and imaging

Sensitivity

For primary or metastatic bone tumors: probably the most sensitive imaging modality except for purely lytic lesions

For infection of vertebrae or disk space: about *85%* [10, 11]

For trauma: nearly *95%* 24 hours after injury [7]

For degenerative disease: high

False negatives can occur
>For infection if process is very aggressive
>Occasionally for trauma in elderly patients [7]
>For tumors that have only small blastic component (e.g., myeloma)

Specificity

For correctly identifying normal area as normal: high
For differentiating among diseases: low—any process causing new bone production will cause an abnormal bone scan

Spine Computed Tomography (CT)

In this setting is particularly useful for evaluating early stages of paravertebral abscesses, infection of epidural space, and spinal cord compression
Illustrates exquisitely the anatomy of facets or processes likely to lead to spinal stenosis

Sensitivity

For early infection: unknown
For late infection: high [2]
For neoplasm: high [4]
For trauma: high [3]
For degenerative disease: high [6]
For processes causing spinal stenosis: high [6, 13]
False negatives can occur
>With early infection
>Occasionally with epidural metastases

Specificity

High, but cannot always differentiate between infection and neoplasm

Metrizamide Myelography

May be more definitive as to presence and location of cord lesion than other tests
Readily available on emergency basis

Drawbacks

Possible side effects: postexamination headache, 62%; nausea and vomiting associated with metrizamide, 38% [1]
Pantopaque use may on rare occasions result in arachnoiditis [8]

Comments

Patient manipulation during myelography may damage spinal cord if spine not stable due to trauma, metastases, etc.

Sensitivity

For localizing cord compression: approaching *100%*

Specificity

Low specificity for cause of cord compression
False positives can occur
> From faulty myelographic technique; injection of contrast into subdural or epidural space instead of subarachnoid space will give the false appearance of tumor or cord compression

Head Computed Tomography (CT)

Identifies potential additional complications of myelography (i.e., brain herniation, spinal cord herniation)
Demonstrates intracranial lesions associated with symptoms and signs of spinal cord compression (see Chap. 30, p. 154 for additional information and data on intracranial masses)

Drawbacks

Potential contrast reactions, 5% (10–12% with history of allergy, 15–16% with previous treatment) [12]

Sensitivity

For intracranial masses: *95%*
For hydrocephalus: approaching *100%*
False negatives can occur
> With lesions having the same attenuation value as surrounding normal brain
> With small lesions adjacent to the bony calvarium

Specificity

For showing normal intracranial structures: high

Contribution of Magnetic Resonance Imaging [9]

Shows spinal anatomy in sagittal and other planes
Fine delineation of normal and abnormal spinal cord
May define edema and necrosis as signals of local disease

References

1. Baker, R. A., Hillman, B. J., McLennan, J. E., et al. Sequelae of metrizamide myelography in 200 examinations. *AJR* 130:499, 1978.
2. Brant-Zawadski, M. Infections. In T. H. Newton and D. G. Potts (Eds.). *Computed Tomography of the Spine and Spinal Cord.* San Anselmo, Cal.: Clavadel Press, 1983. Pp. 205–221.

3. Brant-Zawadski, M., and Post, M. J. D. Trauma. In T. H. Newton and D. G. Potts (Eds.). *Computed Tomography of the Spine and Spinal Cord.* San Anselmo, Cal.: Clavadel Press, 1983. Pp. 149–186.

4. Dorwart, R. H., LaMasters, D. L., and Watanabe, T. J. Tumors. In T. H. Newton and D. G. Potts (Eds.). *Computed Tomography of the Spine and Spinal Cord.* San Anselmo, Cal.: Clavadel Press, 1983. Pp. 115–147.

5. Heinz, E. R. Neuroradiology: Spinal Cord Tumors. In R. N. Rosenberg (Ed.). *The Clinical Neurosciences.* New York: Churchill Livingstone, 1984. Pp. 913–929.

6. Helms, C. A., and Vogler, J. B., III. Spinal Stenosis and Degenerative Lesions. In T. H. Newton and D. G. Potts (Eds.). *Computed Tomography of the Spine and Spinal Cord.* San Anselmo, Cal.: Clavadel Press, 1983. Pp. 251–266.

7. Matin, P. The appearance of bone scans following fractures, including immediate and long term studies. *J. Nucl. Med.* 20:1227, 1978.

8. Mayher, W. E., III, Daniel, E. F., Jr., and Allen, M. B., Jr. Acute meningeal reaction following Pantopaque myelography. *J. Neurosurg.* 34:396, 1971.

9. Norman, D., Mills, C. M., Brant-Zawadzki, M., et al. Magnetic resonance imaging of the spinal cord and canal: Potentials and limitations. *AJNR* 5:9, 1984.

10. Patton, D. D., and Woolfenden, J. M. Radionuclide bone scanning in diseases of the spine. *Radiol. Clin. North Am.* 15:177, 1977.

11. Rodichok, L. D., Harper, G. R., Ruckdeschel, J. C., et al. Early diagnosis of spinal epidural metastases. *Am. J. Med.* 70:1181, 1981.

12. Shehadi, W. H. Contrast media adverse reactions: Occurrence, recurrence and distribution. *Radiology* 143:11, 1982.

13. Williams, A. L., and Haughton, V. M. Disc Herniation and Degenerative Disc Disease. In T. H. Newton and D. G. Potts (Eds.). *Computed Tomography of the Spine and Spinal Cord.* San Anselmo, Cal.: Clavadel Press, 1983. Pp. 231–249.

Thyroid Disease

36

Suspected Thyroid Mass

David E. Drum

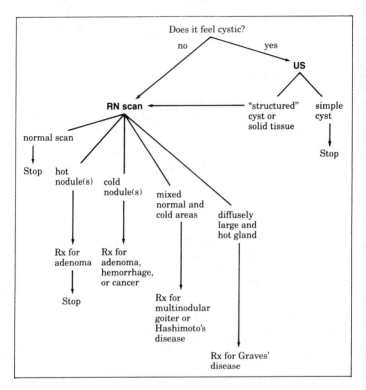

Typical Patient

Individual with suspected thyroid mass based on
    A history of radiation to head, neck, or upper thorax
    A nodule or swelling
    Radiographic evidence of a deviation of the trachea

Typical Disorder(s)

Cancer—malignant or benign tumors
Multinodular goiter
Cyst(s)
Hashimoto's disease
Hemorrhage
Graves' disease

Comments

The major goal of this evaluation is to differentiate benign from
    malignant lesions in the thyroid [9]

This algorithm assumes chemical thyroid function tests are done and the patient is treated appropriately

At some institutions thin needle biopsy is often selected to precede imaging of a palpable nodule. For this approach, it is essential to have both a physician experienced with the biopsy technique and a cytopathologist capable of interpreting reliably the tissue samples obtained [3]

Technetium Pertechnetate Scan

Isotope is trapped but not organified by the thyroid

In general determines whether mass is intrinsic or extrinsic to thyroid and whether the mass is physiologically hyper- or hypoactive [12]

Provides evidence for multicentric disease within thyroid

Can differentiate benign from malignant processes because most tumors will not trap tracer

Drawbacks

Provides no information about adjacent or impinging structures

Thyroid medication or previous contrast studies can affect results: Ideally patient should be off thyroid medication for 4 weeks and have no contrast media for 1 to 2 months

Resolution is limited to detecting nodules about 6 mm in size if pinhole collimator is used

Comments

This algorithm presumes that most tumors will neither trap nor organify pertechnetate or iodide [10]

Nearly 40% of individuals with a single palpable nodule will have multiple nodules by scan [1], thus reducing the probability of cancer to less than 5%

The yield of thyroid carcinoma in patients having a history of neck exposure to radiation *and* a normal neck physical examination is very low (i.e., equal to or less than the prevalence in unselected autopsy examinations)

Iodide as ^{123}I-iodide provides excellent images of low background with intra- or extrathyroidal tissue. Its high cost, lower availability, delay required before imaging, and slightly higher radiation dose generally make [123]I a second choice as radiopharmaceutical

Sensitivity

For suggesting that palpable nodule is malignant: *87–96%*, depending on whether only cold or also cool/warm lesions are considered abnormal [13]

False negatives can occur

    For detection: if nodules are very small

    For calling benign lesions malignant: if tumor traps technetium but not iodide (very rare)

Specificity

For calling benign lesions benign: extremely low, about *15–39%*
[13]
For defining totally normal thyroid tissue as normal: very high
False positives can occur
>   For mass detection: with anomalous lobulations of the thy-
>   roid
>   For misinterpreting benign lesions as potentially malig-
>   nant: in the presence of cysts, adenomas, adenomatous
>   hyperplasia, thyroiditis

Ultrasound (US)

Differentiates cystic from solid lesions
Provides information about adjacent structures [5]

Drawbacks

Provides no functional information

Comments

Recent studies suggest that the prevalence of small (nonpalpa-
ble) benign echogenic "nodules" may be very high (up to 25%)
in patients without clinical suspicion of thyroid disease

Sensitivity

For suggesting that a single palpable nodule is solid or mixed
solid/cystic: *95%* [2, 3, 13]
False negatives can occur
>   With small lesions
>   If thyroid tissue is difficult to identify

Specificity

For calling a purely cystic lesion cystic: approaching *100%* [11],
but purely cystic lesions are very rare

Contribution of Magnetic Resonance Imaging [4, 7]

Readily defines intrathoracic extension of goiter and distinguishes cystic from solid components

References

1. Alderson, P. O., Sumner, H. W., and Siegel, B. A. The single palpable thyroid nodule: Evaluation by ^{99m}Tc-pertechnetate imaging.
   Cancer 37:258, 1976.
2. Ashcraft, M. W., and Van Herle, A. J. Management of thyroid nodules. I: History and physical examination, blood tests, x-ray tests
   and ultrasonography. *Head Neck Surg.* 3:216, 1981.

3. Ashcraft, M. W., and Van Herle, A. J. Management of thyroid nodules. II: Scanning techniques, thyroid suppressive therapy and fine needle aspiration. *Head Neck Surg.* 3:297, 1981.
4. Cohen, A. M., Creviston, S., LiPuma, J. P., et al. NMR evaluation of hilar and mediastinal lymphadenopathy. *Radiology* 148:739, 1983.
5. Cole-Beuglet, C., and Goldberg, B. B. New high-resolution ultrasound evaluation of diseases of the thyroid gland. *JAMA* 249:2941, 1983.
6. DeGroot, L. J., Reilly, M., Pinnameneni, K., et al. Retrospective and prospective study of radiation-induced thyroid disease. *Am. J. Med* 74:852, 1983.
7. Gamsu, G., Stark, D. D., Webb, R., et al. Magnetic resonance imaging of benign mediastinal masses. *Radiology* 151:709, 1984.
8. Maisey, M. N., Moses, D. C., Hurley, P. J., et al. Improved methods for thyroid scanning. A correlation with surgical findings. *JAMA* 223:761, 1973.
9. Mazzaferri, E. L. Solitary thyroid nodule. I. Clinical characteristics. *Postgrad. Med.* 70:98, 1981.
10. Sisson, J. C., Bartold, S. P., and Bartold, S. L. The dilemma of the solitary thyroid nodule: Resolution through decision analysis. *Semin. Nucl. Med.* 8:59, 1978.
11. Spencer, R., Brown, M. C., and Annis, D. Ultrasonic scanning of the thyroid gland as a guide to the treatment of the clinically solitary nodule. *Br. J. Surg.* 64:841, 1977.
12. Task Force on Short-lived Radionuclides for Medical Applications, Bureau of Radiologic Health. Evaluation of diseases of the thyroid gland with the in vivo use of radionuclides. *J. Nucl. Med.* 19:107, 1978.
13. Van Herle, A. J., Rich, P., Ljung, B-M., et al. The thyroid nodule. *Ann. Intern. Med.* 96:221, 1982.
14. Werk, E. E., Vernon, B. M., Gonzalez, J. J., et al. Cancer in thyroid nodules. A community hospital survey. *Arch. Intern. Med.* 144:474, 1984.

VI

Bone Disease

37

Pelvic Trauma, Possible Acetabular Fracture

Barbara N. Weissman

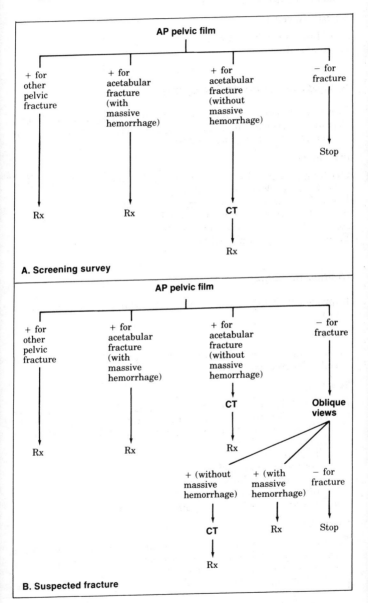

A. Screening survey

B. Suspected fracture

Typical Patient

Individual having a history of severe trauma with or without suspected acetabular injury

Typical Disorder(s)

Acetabular or pelvic fracture
Hip dislocation

Anteroposterior Pelvic Radiography

Provides good general demonstration of anatomy of pelvic bones
Significant overlap makes detection of certain fractures impossible without using other views

Drawbacks

Overlying structures, particularly in the region of the acetabular fossa, make diagnosis difficult
Loose fragments in hip joint may not be seen
Sacral fractures not always defined
Acetabular domes not optimally shown
Fails to identify stable fragment

Oblique Radiograph

Improves visibility of some fracture lines and helps localize others

Drawbacks

Patient must be rolled on hip, causing possible discomfort and risk of increased bleeding

Sensitivity

For AP pelvic view alone or with oblique views: difficult to determine objectively because most studies use CT as truth; sensitivity for fractures is variable, depending on location [1]
   Sacrum/sacroiliac joint: *65–70%*
   Iliac wing: *94%*
   Acetabular roof: *73%*
   Posterior acetabular lip: *88%*
   Pubic rami: approaching *100%*
For detecting loose bodies in joint space: *85%* [1]

Specificity

For AP pelvic view alone or with oblique: difficult to determine objectively because most studies use CT as truth; specificity is variable, depending on location [1]
   Sacrum/sacroiliac joint: *97–100%*
   Iliac wing: *96%*
   Acetabular roof: *93%*

Posterior acetabular lip: *66%*
Pubic rami: approaching *100%*
For differentiating normal joint spaces from those with loose bodies: *89%* [1]

Computed Tomography (CT)

Better than AP and oblique radiographs for detecting intra-articular fracture fragments, femoral head fracture, and hematoma [2, 5, 6, 7, 8]; more information obtained in 50% of acetabular fractures
Defines stable fragment
Can be done in conjunction with other CT examinations

Sensitivity

Currently being used as standard of truth in most studies; data therefore difficult to obtain; however, for detection, it is similar to radiography for iliac wing, anterior and posterior pelvic columns, and pubic rami [1]
More sensitive for detecting fractures than radiography for:
Sacrum/sacroiliac joint: *85–100%*
Iliac wing: *100%*
Acetabular roof: *100%*
Posterior acetabular lip: *97%*
For detecting loose bodies in joints: *98%* [1]
Pubic rami: *100%*
False negatives can occur
If fracture line is parallel to scan plane

Specificity

Currently, by definition for showing bone and joint spaces to be normal in these patients: approaching *100%* [1]
False positives can occur
If partial volume effect superimposes one fracture on another

References

1. Harley, J. D., Mack, L. A., and Winquist, R. A. CT of acetabular fractures: Comparison with conventional radiography. *AJR* 138:413, 1982.
2. Jaeken, R., Casteleyn, P. P., Handelberg, F., et al. Computerized tomography versus conventional radiography in fractures of the acetabulum. *Acta Orthop. Belg.* 48:907, 1982.
3. Judet, R., Judet, J., and Letournel, E. Fractures of the acetabulum: Classification and surgical approaches for open reduction. *J. Bone Joint Surg.* [Am.] 46-A: 1615, 1964.
4. Kane, W. Fractures of the Pelvis. In C. A. Rockwood, Jr., and D. P. Green (Eds.). *Fractures in Adults*. Philadelphia: Lippincott, 1984. Pp. 1093–1209.

5. Rubenstein, J., Kellam, J., and McGonigal, D. Acetabular fracture assessment with computerized tomography. *J. Can. Assoc. Radiol.* 33:139, 1982.
6. Sauser, D. D., Billimoria, P. E., Rouse, G. A., et al. CT evaluation of hip trauma. *AJR* 135:269, 1980.
7. Shirhoda, A., Brashear, H. R., and Staab, E. V. Computed tomography of acetabular fractures. *Radiology* 134:683, 1980.
8. Vas, W. G., Wolverson, M. K., Sundaram, M., et al. The role of computed tomography in pelvic fractures. *J. Comput. Assist. Tomogr.* 6:796, 1982.

Hip Fracture

Piran Aliabadi

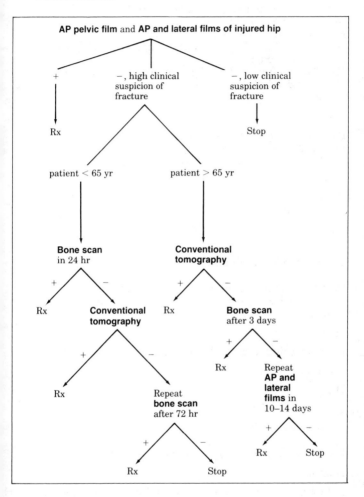

Typical Patient

Elderly individual with osteoporotic bone and history of trauma

Typical Disorder(s)

Intracapsular or extracapsular fracture of femoral neck
Stress fracture
Fracture dislocation

Anteroposterior Pelvic Radiography, Anteroposterior and Lateral Radiography of the Injured Hip

Positive in the majority of patients with fracture
Helps in diagnosis of dislocation
Helps in exclusion of articular disease
Helps to evaluate bones for other underlying diseases such as metastasis, Paget's
10–14 days after fracture, bone resorption at the fracture margins and additional radiographic signs of healing are frequently seen

Sensitivity

For diagnosing fractures: high
False negatives can occur
    With overlapping structures

Specificity

High
False positives can occur
    In the presence of osteophytes

Conventional Tomography

Conventional tomography in AP projection can help in diagnosing some fractures that are not originally diagnosed by plain films

Sensitivity

For diagnosing fracture: higher than that of plain films

Specificity

High

Bone Scan

Useful for diagnosing stress fracture and occult fracture

Drawbacks

2- to 4-hour delay required between injection of radiotrace and imaging
As much as 24–72 hours may be needed for scintigram to become abnormal (some cases are positive within hours after fracture)

Sensitivity

For all ages 24 hours after fracture: *80%*; under age 65: *95%* [3, 4, 6]

For all ages 3 days after fracture: *95%*; under age 65: *100%* [3, 4, 6]

For all ages 1 week after fracture: *98%*; under age 65: *100%* [3, 4, 6]

Specificity

No data available, but probably low

False positives may occur

> In the presence of soft tissue injury, infection, metastasis, inflammatory arthritis, and healed fracture

References

1. Felson, B. *Roentgenology of Fractures and Dislocations.* New York: Grune & Stratton, 1978.
2. Harris, J. H., and Harris, W. H. *The Radiology of Emergency Medicine* (2nd ed.). Baltimore: Williams & Wilkins, 1984.
3. Matin, P. The appearance of bone scans following fractures, including immediate and long-term studies. *J. Nucl. Med.* 20:1227, 1979.
4. Matin, P. Bone scintigraphy in the diagnosis and management of traumatic injury. *Semin. Nucl. Med.* 13:104, 1983.
5. Resnick, D., and Niwayama, G. *Diagnosis of Bone and Joint Disorders.* Philadelphia: Saunders, 1981.
6. Rosenthall, L., Hill, R., and Chuang, S. Observation on the use of ^{99m}Tc-phosphate imaging in peripheral bone trauma. *Radiology* 119:637, 1976.

High Clinical Suspicion of Fracture of a Long Bone

Vera L. Stewart

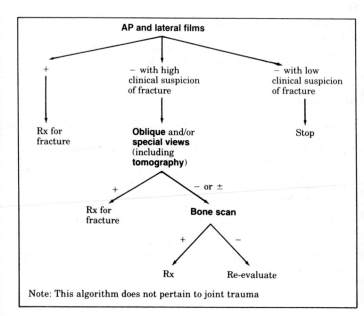

Note: This algorithm does not pertain to joint trauma

Typical Patient

Individual who experienced trauma and has ecchymoses, crepitation, soft tissue swelling, point tenderness, bony deformity, or instability [2, 3]

Typical Disorder(s)

Acute fractures
Stress fractures
Soft tissue trauma

Plain Films

Allows identification of fracture site
Allows assessment of alignment of fragments
Diagnostic for most patients after initial films

Drawbacks

Sometimes requires follow-up film for stress fracture without displacement or separation

Sensitivity

No specific data available for diagnosing acute traumatic fracture, but usually high; for stress fracture, high

Specificity

No data available

Tomography

Particularly at the knee, allows identification of fracture in osteoporotic patients [1]
More sensitive than plain films

Drawbacks

Sometimes requires follow-up for stress fracture without displacement or separation

Sensitivity

No specific data available, but for diagnosing fracture, very high

Specificity

No data available, but usually very high

Bone Scan

Evaluates acute trauma, multiple trauma, stress and occult fractures

Comment

Should be done at least 6 hours after trauma

Sensitivity

Age dependent: less than 65 years old, *98%*; over 65, *95%* [4]
False negatives can occur
    If scan is done too quickly after fracture

Specificity

No data available, but in previously normal bone likely to be high

References

1. Apple, J. S., Martinez, S., Allen, N. B., et al. Occult fractures of the knee: Tomographic evaluation. *Radiology* 148:383, 1983.
2. Brand, D. A., Frazier, W. H., Kohlhepp, W. C., et al. A protocol for selecting patients with injured extremities who need x-rays. *N. Engl. J. Med.* 306:333, 1982.

3. de Lacey, G., and Bradbrooke, S. Rationalising requests for x-ray examination of acute ankle injuries. *Br. Med. J.* 1:1597, 1979.
4. Matin, P. Bone scintigraphy in the diagnosis and management of traumatic injury. *Semin. Nucl. Med.* 13:104, 1983.,

Clinical Suspicion of Nonunion

Vera L. Stewart

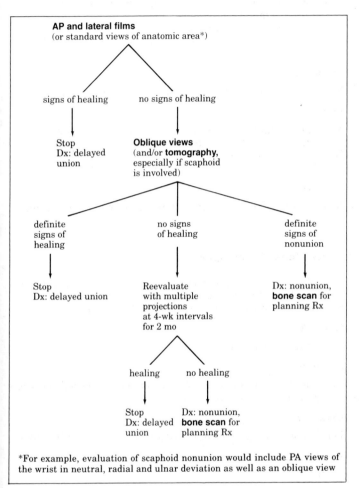

*For example, evaluation of scaphoid nonunion would include PA views of the wrist in neutral, radial and ulnar deviation as well as an oblique view

Typical Patient

Individual with treated and observed fractures experiencing pain and having clinical evidence of motion, suspicion of infection or delayed healing

Typical Disorder(s)

Nonunion
Delayed union
Malunion

Plain Film

Affords assessment of bone healing and permits the diagnosis of osteonecrosis, infection, cystic degeneration, displacement of fracture fragments, or abnormal motion about fracture site
AP and lateral views: illustrate healing process
Oblique view: increases probability of observing minimal callus formation

Drawbacks

Not always possible to distinguish infection from nonunion

Sensitivity

No data available but likely to be high: Radiographs are very sensitive for evidence of the healing process per se
False negatives can occur
  If fracture line cannot be visualized in profile

Specificity

No data available but likely high (specificity likely to be higher than sensitivity)

Conventional Tomography

Clarifies the anatomical characteristics of the region of interest when plain films are not adequate for evaluation
Eliminates confusion due to overlying structures

Drawbacks

Higher radiation dose

Comments

Computed tomography can be considered in special locations (e.g., pelvic or spine fractures)

Sensitivity

For demonstrating signs of nonunion or signs of healing: high

Specificity

High

Bone Scan

Major role is not for diagnosis; rather, it is used for treatment planning, that is, to document pseudoarthrosis (as manifested by central cold area between adjacent areas of increased uptake) [2, 3]

Sensitivity/Specificity

There are few published articles on the value of bone scans in predicting the response to percutaneous electrical stimulation; for example, see reference 3. Results in this context are best summarized in terms of predictive values rather than of sensitivities and specificities.

When there is no cold "gap" seen on bone scan, *94%* of patients will heal on percutaneous electrical stimulation.

When a cold gap is seen, a much smaller percentage (less than *20%*) will heal.

False negatives can occur if cold gap is incorrectly missed because of

Poor resolution, particularly if fractures involve small bones

Presence of a cast, precluding good examination

Poor technique, that is, inadequate views

Superimposed infection

References

1. Brighton, C. T. Treatment of nonunion of the tibia with constant direct current (1980 Fitts Lecture, A.A.S.T.). *J. Trauma* 21:189, 1981.
2. Desai, A., Alavi, A., Dalinka, M., et al. Role of bone scintigraphy in the evaluation and treatment of nonunited fractures: Concise communication. *J. Nucl. Med.* 21:931, 1980.
3. Esterhal, J. L., Jr., Brighton, C. T., Heppenstall, R. B., et al. Detection of synovial pseudoarthrosis by ^{99m}Tc scintigraphy: Application to treatment of traumatic nonunion with constant direct current. *Clin. Orthop. Rel. Res.* 161:15, 1981.
4. Naimark, A., Miller, K., Segal, D., et al. Nonunion. *Skeletal Radiol.* 6:21, 1981.
5. Wilson, J. N. United Fractures and the Transplantation of Bone. In R. Watson-Jones (Ed.). *Fractures and Joint Injuries.* New York: Churchill Livingstone, 1982. Pp. 436–465, 482–483.

Osteonecrosis

George F. Edeburn and Sabah S. Tumeh

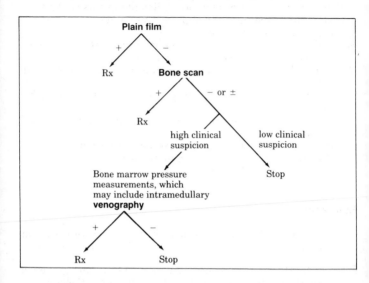

Typical Patient

Individuals who have had trauma to bone

Nontraumatized individuals with high risk pre-existing disease state including steroid therapy, alcoholism, pancreatitis, hemoglobinopathies, gout, Gaucher's disease, and Caisson's disease

Typical Disorder(s)

Osteonecrosis
Arthritis
Degenerative disease

Comments

Early diagnosis is considered important because early detection with early therapy (reduction in weight bearing, surgical decompression) may prevent progression leading to collapse of articular cartilage

Intraosseous cannulation with bone marrow pressure measurements (frequently including intramedullary venography) is used as basis for gold standard and for definitive diagnosis. Pressures over 30 mm Hg approach *100%* in sensitivity; associated specificities also approach *100%* [3].

Plain Film

Plain film changes, when present, are characteristics of osteonecrosis

Early radiographic changes include patchy lucent areas and osteoporosis with the subsequent appearance of an arclike sub-
chondral lucency [6]. The latter finding represents the so-
called crescent sign.

Later changes include collapse or flattening and subsequently,
in joints, changes suggestive of osteoarthritis [6]

Drawbacks

Radiographic changes are often not present until months after
the onset of symptoms

Sensitivity

Few data; however, for detecting osteonecrosis in asymptomatic
patients being treated with steroids for systemic lupus erythematosus: *50%* [1]

False negatives can occur if disease is very early

Specificity

No data available but early in the course of disease radiographic
changes are characteristic and the specificity should be very
high

Later in the course of disease arthritides may cause confusion
in interpretation

Bone Scan

Very sensitive to the presence of osteonecrosis

Early: In the first few weeks after the vascular insult, the impaired vascular supply will result in decreased uptake [2]

Late: During the revascularization and reparative process, the
bone scan will show increased uptake [2]

Pinhole views are usually required

Companion radiographs may be necessary for interpretation

Drawbacks

Early cold lesions may be missed if very small

Lesion may be masked by other osseous disorders (e.g., arthritides)

Sensitivity

Few data; however, for detecting osteonecrosis in asymptomatic
patients being treated with steroids for systemic lupus erythematosus: *77%* [1]

For detecting osteonecrosis in symptomatic patients being
treated with steroids for systemic lupus erythematosus: approaching *100%* [1]

False negatives can occur in presence of
    Early disease
    Small cold lesion
    Suboptimal scanning technique because
        Pinhole views were not obtained
        There is high background activity (e.g., renal failure)

Specificity

No data available but likely to be high
False positives can occur in presence of
    Other osseous abnormality
    Suboptimal scanning techniques, particularly caused by high bladder activity

Venography

Usually performed at the same time as bone marrow pressure recording
Intramedullary venography demonstrating poor filling of extraosseous veins, diaphyseal reflux, and delayed clearance of contrast material is evidence of osteonecrosis [1, 3, 5]

Drawbacks

Invasive—requires placement of intramedullary needle
Uncomfortable—requires sedation and/or anesthesia
Occasionally (6%) technically inadequate [5]

Sensitivity

No data available but high; in one study a 92% correlation of venography with tetracycline evaluation of head viability was found [5]

Specificity

No data available, but high if filling of extraosseous veins is seen [3, 5]

Contribution of Magnetic Resonance Imaging [4, 7]

Recent studies suggest that MRI may identify ischemic necrosis of the femoral head better than CT or radionuclide tests

References

1. Conklin, J. J., Alderson, P. O., Zizic, T. M., et al. Comparison of bone scan and radiograph sensitivity in the detection of steroid induced ischemic necrosis of bone. *Radiology* 147:221, 1983.
2. D'Ambrosia, R. D., Shoji, H., Riggins, R. S., et al. Scintigraphy in the diagnosis of osteonecrosis. *Clin. Orthop. Rel. Res.* 130:139, 1978.

3. Hungerford, D. S. Early diagnosis of ischemic necrosis of the femoral head. *Johns Hopkins Med. J.* 137:270, 1975.
4. Moon, K. L., Genant, H. K., Helms, C. A., et al. Musculoskeletal application of nuclear magnetic resonance. *Radiology* 147:161, 1983.
5. Outerbridge, R. E. Perosseous venography in the diagnosis of viability in subcapital fractures of the femur. *Clin. Orthop. Rel. Res.* 137:132, 1978.
6. Resnick, D., and Niwayama, G. In *Diagnosis of Bone and Joint Disease,* Vol. 3. Philadelphia: Saunders, 1981. Pp. 2835–2840.
7. Totty, W. G., Murphy, W. A., Ganz, W. I., et al. Magnetic resonance imaging of the normal and ischemic femoral head. *AJR* 143:1273, 1984.

42

Total Hip Replacement, Associated Pain

Barbara N. Weissman

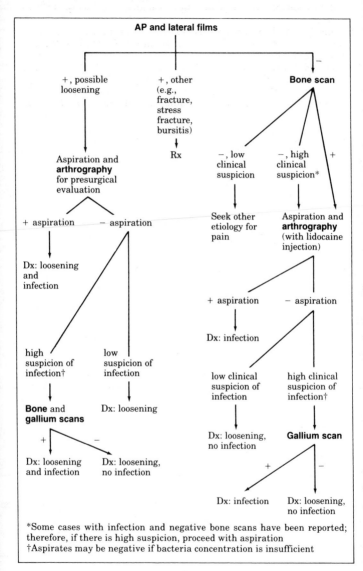

*Some cases with infection and negative bone scans have been reported; therefore, if there is high suspicion, proceed with aspiration
†Aspirates may be negative if bacteria concentration is insufficient

Typical Patient

Individual with total hip replacement experiencing pain

Typical Disorder(s)

Loosening, infection, loosening with infection
Stress fractures
Dislocations
Bursitis
Referred pain

Plain Films (AP and Lateral)

Help exclude periarticular disease (e.g., fracture or trochanteric bursitis)
Help evaluate loosening but cannot diagnose superimposed infection
Necessary prior to other procedures

Sensitivity

For prostheses with opaque cement:
    For loosening of acetabular component: *93%* [7, 14]
    For loosening of femoral component: *91%* [7, 14]
    For infection at any site: *50%* [14]
False negatives can occur for prostheses with either opaque or nonopaque cement
    If infection is present without loosening

Specificity

For distinguishing normal from either loosening or infection at any site: *91%* [7, 14]
For distinguishing normal from loosening of acetabular component: *84%* [7, 14]
For distinguishing normal from loosening of femoral component: approaching *100%* [7, 14]

Bone Scan

Useful for detecting loosening and/or infection

Drawbacks

May not be able to distinguish loosening from infection; however, focal rather than diffuse uptake is more indicative of aseptic loosening than infection [15]
Unreliable within the first 6–10 months following surgery because increased uptake normally exists during that time

Sensitivity

For loosening alone at acetabular component: *80%* [7, 14]
For loosening alone at femoral component: *97%* [7, 14]
For infection at any site: published literature suggests values approaching *100%* [14, 15, 17]; unpublished data, considerably lower [1]

False negatives can occur

Because of the difficulty in distinguishing ectopic bone from loosening/infection of the acetabular component, readers hesitate to diagnose abnormalities in this area: thus, decreased sensitivity and increased specificity

Specificity

For distinguishing normal from either loosening or infection in the acetabular region: *90%* [7, 14, 15, 17]

For distinguishing normal from either loosening or infection in the femoral region: *70%* [7, 14, 15, 17]

False positives can occur

From ectopic bone causing increased uptake

Joint Aspiration for Culture, Cell Count, Smear

Provides direct sampling of joint fluid [9]

Drawbacks

May be uncomfortable
Rare infection introduced

Sensitivity

Over *80%* [3]

False negatives can occur with

An insufficient quantity of bacteria
An inability to aspirate joint fluid
Inadequate cultures obtained

Specificity

85–100%

False positives can occur

If sample is contaminated (up to 15%)

Arthrography

Confirms intra-articular needle position for fluid aspiration, may confirm loosening, may suggest infection [6]

After cultures have been obtained, lidocaine can be instilled into the joint. The absence of pain after this injection accurately localizes pain to the hip (rather than to periarticular structures) [3].

Drawbacks

May be uncomfortable

Sensitivity

For loosening of acetabular component: *59%* [14, 17]
For loosening of femoral component: *67%* [14, 17]

False negatives can occur
>   If low volume of contrast or low pressure injections are used; high pressure techniques increase sensitivity at both components to *95%* [8]

Specificity

For distinguishing normal acetabular component from loosening: *83%* [14, 17]

For distinguishing normal femoral component from loosening: approaching *100%* [14, 17]

False positives can occur [10]
>   Depending on definition of loosening used: Radiographic evidence of abnormal bond at prosthesis-cement or cement-bone interfaces does not always correspond to physically loose prothesis at surgery

Gallium Scan

Thought by some to have high sensitivity and specificity, particularly for active, untreated, bacterial infection

However, data on its use are controversial: One study [11] suggests high accuracy; recent unpublished data [1] do not support this

Drawbacks

Must compare to bone scan

Sensitivity

For detecting infection: May be as low as *50%* [1]
or nearly *100%* [11, 16]

Specificity

With conservative criteria for interpreting bone and gallium results: probably high [11]

References

1. Aliabadi, P., Tumeh, S. S., Weissman, B. N., et al. Radiologic Evaluation of Total Joint Prostheses (unpublished data, RSNA, 1985)
2. Anderson, L. S., and Staple, T. N. Arthrography of total hip replacement using subtraction technique. *Radiology* 109:470, 1973.
3. Burton, D. S., Propst-Proctor, S. L., and Schurman, D. J. Anesthetic hip arthrography in the diagnosis of postoperative hip pathology. *Contemp. Orthop.* 7:17, 1983.
4. Dussault, R. G., Goldman, A. B., and Ghelman, B. Radiologic diagnosis of loosening and infection in hip prostheses. *J. Can. Assoc. Radiol.* 28:119, 1977.
5. Firooznia, H., Baruch, H., Seliger, G., et al. The value of subtraction in hip arthrography after total hip replacement. *Bull. Hosp. Joint Dis.* 35:36, 1974.

6. Gelman, M. I. Arthrography in total hip prosthesis complications. *AJR* 126:743, 1976.

7. Gelman, M. I., Coleman, R. E., Stevens, P. M., et al. Radiography, radionuclide imaging, and arthrography in the evaluation of total hip and knee replacement. *Radiology* 128:677, 1978.

8. Hendrix, R. W., Wixson, R. L., Rana, N. A., et al. Arthrography after total hip arthroplasty: A modified technique used in the diagnosis of pain. *Radiology* 148:647, 1983.

9. McLaughlin, R. E., and Whitehill, R. Evaluation of the painful hip by aspiration and arthrography. *Surg. Gynecol. Obstet.* 144:381, 1977.

10. Murray, W. R., and Rodrigo, J. J. Arthrography for the assessment of pain after total hip replacement. A comparison of arthrographic findings in patients with and without pain. *J. Bone Joint Surg.* 57A:1060, 1975.

11. Rosenthall, L., Lisbona, R., Hernandez, M., et al. ^{99m}Tc-PP and ^{67}Ga imaging following insertion of orthopedic devices. *Radiology* 133:717, 1979.

12. Salvati, E. A., Freiberger, R. H., and Wilson, P. D. Arthrography for complications of total hip replacement. A review of thirty-one arthrograms. *J. Bone Joint Surg.* 53A:701, 1971.

13. Salvati, E. A., Ghelman, B., McLaren, T., et al. Subtraction technique in arthrography for loosening of total hip replacement fixed with radiopaque cement. *Clin. Orthop.* 101:103, 1974.

14. Tehranzadeh, J., Schneider, R., Freiberger, R. H. Radiological evaluation of painful total hip replacement. *Radiology* 141:355, 1981.

15. Weiss, P. E., Mall, J. C., Hoffer, P. B., et al. ^{99m}Tc-methylene diphosphonate bone imaging in the evaluation of total hip prostheses. *Radiology* 133:727, 1979.

16. Williams, F., McCall, I. W., Park, W. M., et al. Gallium-67 scanning in the painful total hip replacement. *Clin. Radiol.* 32:431, 1981.

17. Williamson, B. R. J., McLaughlin, R. E., Wang, G.-J., et al. Radionuclide bone imaging as a means of differentiating loosening and infection in patients with a painful total hip prosthesis. *Radiology* 133:723, 1979.

43

Osteomyelitis

Sabah S. Tumeh

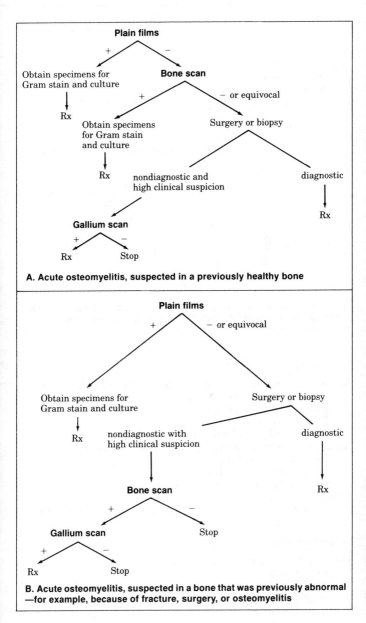

A. Acute osteomyelitis, suspected in a previously healthy bone

B. Acute osteomyelitis, suspected in a bone that was previously abnormal —for example, because of fracture, surgery, or osteomyelitis

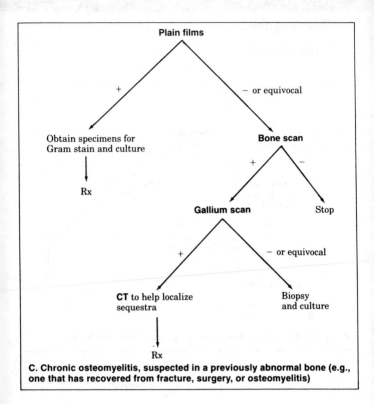

C. Chronic osteomyelitis, suspected in a previously abnormal bone (e.g., one that has recovered from fracture, surgery, or osteomyelitis)

Typical Patient

Acute osteomyelitis in patient with previously healthy bone
    Child with *Staphylococcus aureus*
    Individual with septicemia
    IV drug addicts
    Elderly individual with UTI, diabetes
Acute osteomyelitis in patient with abnormal bone
    Individual with previous orthopedic surgery
    Individual with fractures
    Individual with sickle cell disease
Chronic osteomyelitis
    Individual with prior bone infection with suspected exacerbation

Typical Disorder(s)

Bone/joint disorders
    Bone infection
    Arthritides
    Bone infarct
    Bone tumor

Soft tissue disease
    Cellulitis
    Soft tissue abscess

Plain Films

May show periosteal reaction, erosions, or sequestra and make
the diagnosis quickly

Drawbacks

Changes may be nonspecific because other diseases may mimic
the radiological changes

Sensitivity

In children: very low, particularly during first 2 weeks
In adults: low [9], especially in presence of previous bone disease
False negatives can occur
    In children: because of early disease (first week)

Specificity

In children: very high
In adults: very low
False positives can occur
    In children: Other permeative lesions may have similar ra-
        diographic appearance (e.g., leukemia, Ewing's sarcoma)
    In adults: because of previous bone disease with sclerosis
        and periosteal reaction (e.g., inactive osteomyelitis, pre-
        vious fractures or surgery)

Bone Scan

Very sensitive to site and presence of disease, particularly acute
disease
Companion radiographs are necessary for interpretation

Drawbacks

Relatively nonspecific, particularly in patients with previous or
other bone disease (e.g., patient with pain, negative radiograph, positive bone scan, who turns out to have a fracture or
infarct)
Increased specificity may require concomitant gallium scans, especially in algorithm B where surgery may have been done
prior to bone scanning; these may delay interpretation by 48
hours
Occasionally difficult to differentiate soft tissue disease from adjacent osteomyelitis; multiple views or tomography may facil-
itate this differentiation

Comments

Equivocal studies occur primarily in children; increased uptake in the metaphysis adjacent to the epiphysis may not be distinguishable from epiphyseal activity per se

Emergency bone scan indicated in acute hematogenous osteomyelitis with negative plain films

Sensitivity

In children: about *84%* [3, 6, 7]

In adults: considerably higher, probably close to *100%* [4, 5, 7, 9]

False negatives can occur with

   Early aggressive (difference in sensitivities between children and adults may reflect the earliness of diagnosis)

   Vascular insufficiency

Specificity

For showing normal bone without evidence of osteomyelitis: about *92%* [3]

At sites of previous disease, for differentiating active from inactive disease: low, only *20–30%* [5, 6, 9]

False positives can occur with

   Hyperemia

   Fractures

   Prior surgery

   Bone infarcts

   Inactive disease

   Arthropathies

   Tumors

   Disuse osteoporesis

Gallium Scan

More specific than bone scans

Useful in differentiating active from inactive disease

May be helpful in defining anatomical extent of infection and areas that require debridement

Drawbacks

Requires 24–48 hours between injection and imaging

Requires complicated interpretation scheme; probability of osteomyelitis depends on degree and extent of gallium uptake

A negative gallium scan cannot differentiate between dormant infection and cured disease

Sensitivity

In children: probably close to *100%* (i.e., all children with osteomyelitis have either abnormal bone and/or gallium scans)

In adults: somewhat lower and controversial: some values as high as *100%* [5, 6]; others about *90%* [9]

False negatives can occur

With fungal infections

Possibly with associated long courses of intravenous antibiotic therapy

With infections due to indolent bacteria

Specificity

For showing normal bone in areas without previous bone disease: very high, approaching *100%*

For differentiating active from dormant or cured previous disease: somewhat lower and variable depending on criteria used to interpret gallium studies

As with the diagnosis of pulmonary embolism (see p. 125), multiple bone/gallium scan patterns are possible, and the chance of osteomyelitis varies with these patterns [9]. For example:

If gallium uptake exceeds bone uptake, probability is close to *100%*

If the bone uptake is considerably greater than the gallium uptake, the probability is about *14%*

If there is gallium activity outside the region of the bone activity, the probability is about *78%*

False positives can occur with

Bowel activity (if pelvis is involved)

Active inflammatory processes (e.g., arthritides)

Tumors (e.g., synovial cell sarcoma)

Fractures

Computed Tomography (CT)

Most useful in suspected chronic osteomyelitis: in planning for surgery, defining soft tissue collection(s) that need drainage

Broad dynamic range permits viewing both bone and soft tissues

Combines excellent contrast resolution with good spatial resolution

Can map extent of disease for possible surgical intervention (e.g., finding sequestra)

Drawbacks

Requires companion radiographs, bone scans, or localizing device (scoutview) for accurate mapping of area of concern and for proper interpretation

In general only a limited area of the skeleton can be examined

May offer too much information (e.g., clinically unimportant soft tissue masses may be diagnosed as abscesses in patients with spinal osteomyelitis)

Sensitivity

For detecting osteomyelitis: no data but probably higher than plain films and lower than bone scans

False negatives can occur
>   From motion
>   From surgical clips or devices
>   With early disease

Specificity

For showing normal bone as normal: no data, but probably high
For differentiating among causes of disease in previously abnormal bone: moderate
False positives can occur
>   If sclerosis is mistaken for sequestra

Contribution of Magnetic Resonance Imaging [1, 2, 8]

May demonstrate acute osteomyelitis early: shows involvement of soft tissues
Its potential for distinguishing inflammation from malignancy is uncertain

References

1. Berquist, T. H. Preliminary experience in orthopedic radiology. *Magnetic Resonance Imaging* 2:41, 1984.
2. Fletcher, B. D., Scoles, P. V., and Nelson, A. D. Osteomyelitis in children: Detection by magnetic resonance. *Radiology* 150:57, 1984.
3. Gelfand, M. J., and Silberstein, E. B. Radionuclide imaging use in diagnosis of osteomyelitis in children. *JAMA* 237:245, 1977.
4. Hoffer, P. Gallium and infection. *J. Nucl. Med.* 21:484, 1980.
5. Lisbona, R., and Rosenthall, L. Observations on the sequential use of ^{99m}Tc-phosphate complex and ^{67}Ga imaging in osteomyelitis, cellulitis and septic arthritis. *Radiology* 123:123, 1977.
6. Lisbona, R., and Rosenthall, L. Radionuclide imaging of septic joints and their differentiation from periarticular osteomyelitis and cellulitis in pediatrics. *Clin. Nucl. Med.* 2:337, 1977.
7. Markisz, J. A., and McNeil, B. J. Bone Remodeling. In P. O. Alderson (Ed.). *Nuclear Radiology* (3rd series), syllabus. Chicago: American College of Radiology, 1983. Pp. 476–491.
8. Smith, F. W., Runge, V., Permezel, M., et al. Nuclear magnetic resonance (NMR) imaging in the diagnosis of spinal osteomyelitis. *Magnetic Resonance Imaging* 2:53, 1984.
9. Tumeh, S. S., Aliabadi, P., Weissman, B. N., et al. Abnormal Tc 99m/Ga-67 scan patterns in association with active chronic osteomyelitis (abstract). *J. Nucl. Med.* 26:24, 1985.

44

Osteoporosis

J. Leland Sosman

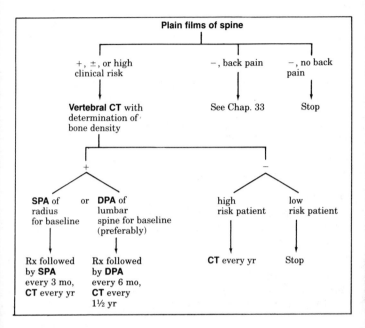

Typical Patients

Individuals experiencing back pain, with or without trauma, especially women at or after menopause

Asymptomatic high risk patients (e.g., corticosteroid recipient)

Typical Disorder(s)

Deficient cancellous bone in axial skeleton

Plain Films of Spine

Excellent demonstration of gross anatomy

Clear delineation of gross osteoporosis

Provides localization for special examinations

Drawbacks

Poor accuracy; relatively subjective, hence operator dependent

Insensitive until disease is well advanced

Sensitivity

About 60%, but the number is difficult to obtain because there is no good calibration endpoint except for fractures

Specificity

Approaching *100%* in the absence of osteomalacia or diffuse malignancy (e.g., multiple myeloma)
False positives can occur
    In the presence of osteomalacia or diffuse malignancy
    With residual vertebral wedging from previous Scheuermann's juvenile apophysitis

Vertebral Computed Tomography (CT) (with Included Reference Phantom and Computer Evaluation)

Measures cancellous bone at the site of maximum risk
Measurements are good for longitudinal studies

Drawbacks

Expensive and not universally available

Sensitivity

No exact data available, but high for cancellous bone: For example, cancellous site measurements are 5 times as sensitive as cortical sites [2]

Specificity

Approaching *100%*
False positives can occur
    In the presence of osteomalacia

Dual Photon Absorptiometry (DPA)

Use of two pulse height analyzers helps eliminate the effect of soft tissue on absorption measurements
Primarily used for measurements of the lumbar spine and axial bone density
Delivers a lower radiation dose than CT: Peak skin dose is less than 20 mrad [5]

Drawbacks

Can be used in AP projection only
Measurements are the sum of cortical and cancellous (trabecular) bone and include posterior spinal elements
Soft tissue calcification, osteophytes, and callus can influence results
Metallic orthopedic devices or metallic objects on clothing can lead to uninterpretable results

Sensitivity

No precise data, but considerably more sensitive than single photon absorptiometry, but less sensitive than CT, which can limit measurements to only cancellous bone components

False negatives can occur with
   Soft tissue calcifications
   Osteophytes
   Callus
   Many other focal spinal processes (e.g., Paget's disease)

Specificity

Approaching *100%*
False positives can occur
   In the presence of osteomalacia

Single Photon Absorptiometry (SPA) (Wrist or Distal Radius)

Useful for sequential studies
Rapid, comfortable, noninvasive, inexpensive

Drawbacks

Density of wrist is not necessarily parallel to osteoporosis of spine [6]
Does not measure bone density in area of critical interest, namely the spine
Partially to largely subject to cortical bone density component (depending on site scanned)

Sensitivity

About *85%*; however, for most classes of patients predictive value of axial bone loss is low, only *50–60%*
False negatives can occur if
   Peripheral skeleton is within normal density limits while axial skeleton is below normal density (particularly in early or developing cases, in osteoporosis accompanying steroids or alcohol, or in male idiopathic osteoporosis)

Specificity

Approaching *100%*
False positives can occur
   In the presence of osteomalacia

References

1. Cann, C. E., and Genant, H. K. Precise measurement of vertebral mineral content using computed tomography. *J. Comput. Assist. Tomogr.* 4:493, 1980.
2. Genant, H. K., Cann, C. E., and Boyd, D. O. Quantitative Computed Tomography for Vertebral Mineral Determination. In B. Frame and J. T. Potts (Eds.). *Clinical Disorders of Bone and Mineral Metabolism.* New York: Excerpta Medica, 1983. Pp. 40–47.

3. Kovarik, J., Küster, W., Seidl, G., et al. Clinical relevance of radiologic examination of the skeleton and bone density measurements in osteoporosis of old age. *Skeletal Radiol.* 7:37, 1981.
4. Sandor, T., Weissman, B., Hanlon, W. B., et al. Assessment of mineral changes in the spine with computer tomography using a calibration phantom. Application of Optical Instrumentation in Medicine XII. *SPIE* 454:192, 1984.
5. Wahner, H. W., Dunn, W. L., and Riggs, B. L. Assessment of bone mineral. *J. Nucl. Med.* 25:1134, 1241, 1984.
6. Wilson, C. R. Bone-mineral content of the femoral neck and spine versus the radius or ulna. *J. Bone Joint Surg.* 59A:665, 1977.

Peripheral Vascular Disease

Acute Leg Pain of Suspected Vascular Origin

Michael A. Bettmann

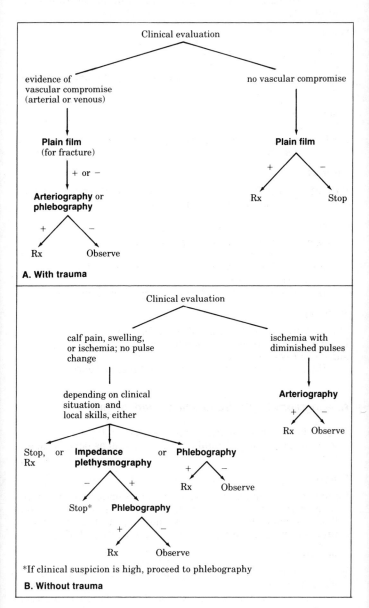

A. With trauma

Clinical evaluation

evidence of vascular compromise (arterial or venous)

Plain film (for fracture)

+ or −

Arteriography or phlebography

+ −

Rx   Observe

no vascular compromise

Plain film

+ −

Rx   Stop

B. Without trauma

Clinical evaluation

calf pain, swelling, or ischemia; no pulse change

depending on clinical situation and local skills, either

Stop, or **Impedance** or **Phlebography** Rx **plethysmography**

+ −

Rx   Observe

− +

Stop* **Phlebography**

+ −

Rx   Observe

ischemia with diminished pulses

Arteriography

+ −

Rx   Observe

*If clinical suspicion is high, proceed to phlebography

Typical Patient

Individual experiencing pain, whether associated with trauma or not, thought to be vascular in origin, in any portion of one or both legs

Typical Disorder(s)

Arterial trauma or occlusion
Deep or superficial venous thrombosis
Chronic arterial or venous disease, with superimposed process

Plain Films

Useful in guiding further evaluation whether results are positive or negative

Comment

Patients suspected of bone or soft tissue pathology might require other diagnostic examinations

Sensitivity

Varies widely with underlying pathology
    For fracture: high
    For vascular and most soft tissue processes: low
False negatives can occur
    In the presence of soft tissue or vascular pathology

Specificity

For fracture: high (and generally sufficient)
For most other processes: not specific
False positives can occur
    Rarely, from misinterpretation and inexperience

Arteriography/Digital Subtraction Arteriography

Generally answers specific questions accurately
Useful for diagnosing thrombi in aorta as well as peripheral emboli

Drawbacks

Complications: contrast reaction and/or secondary renal failure, rare (more common in diabetics); vascular injury and thrombosis, serious, about 1%; local hemorrhage or hematoma, nonfatal serious reactions, less than 2%; fatalities, .03% [6]

Comments

Resolution of standard arteriography is superior to that of digital subtraction
Digital subtraction is less invasive and is used more as a screening test

Improved contrast agents are decreasing possible contrast-related complications

Mural thrombi in aorta pose risk for dislodgment and embolization to viscera or legs [11]

Sensitivity

For most applications (e.g., arterial occlusion): high
For mural thrombi of aorta leading to peripheral thrombi: high [11]
False negatives can occur
    From poor technique

Specificity

In skilled hands, can exceed *95%*
False positives can occur
    From poor technique
    With spasm

Lower Limb Phlebography

Properly performed, is highly accurate in detecting venous thrombosis

Drawbacks

Not a screening procedure
Overall complication rate: 3% with standard contrast agents, 0% with new nonionic agents (postphlebography phlebitis) [2]

Comments

Although radiation exposure is not high, the examination is relatively contraindicated for pregnant patients

Sensitivity

Commonly used as the gold standard; for detecting thrombi larger than 0.5 cm, approaching *100%*
False negatives can occur
    If patient does not relax leg
    From poor technique
    From careless interpretation or failure to delineate major veins

Specificity

95% if strict criteria are used (intraluminal filling defect in more than one view); lower with less rigid technique and interpretation
False positives can occur
    With less rigid interpretative criteria (e.g., lack of visualization of a vein or gradual cut-off)

Impedance Plethysmography

Noninvasive and can be performed at bedside; can be repeated
   as often as needed

Drawbacks

Insensitive to calf thrombi
Requires expertise and experience to perform and interpret,
   with large range in reported values for sensitivity (*30–100%*)
   and specificity (*19–100%*) [10]

Comments

Extremity must be flexible, not in a cast, and the patient must
   cooperate

Sensitivity

Overall average: *90%* [10], with *90–95%* for acute proximal
   thrombi and less than *65%* for distal thrombi
False negatives can occur
   With small or even large nonocclusive or distal thrombi that
      do not alter blood flow

Specificity

For showing normal vessels: about *90%* [10]
False positives can occur
   From alterations in lower extremity venous volume or flow
      (e.g., pregnancy, abdominal mass, right heart failure,
      muscle contraction)

Contribution of Magnetic Resonance Imaging [4, 5]

May demonstrate vascular anatomy, blood flow, intraluminal
   thrombus, vascular occlusion

References

1. Baum, S., Stein, G. N., and Kuroda, K. K. Complications of "no
   arteriography." *Radiology* 86:835, 1966.
2. Bettmann, M. A., Salzman, E. W., Rosenthal, D., et al. Reduction
   of venous thrombosis complicating phlebography. *AJR* 134:1169,
   1980.
3. Formanek, G., Frech, R. S., and Amplatz, K. Arterial thrombus
   formation during clinical percutaneous catheterization. *Circulation* 41:833, 1970.
4. Herfkens, R. J., Higgins, C. B., Hricak, H., et al. Nuclear magnetic
   resonance imaging of the cardiovascular system: Normal and
   pathologic findings. *Radiology* 147:749, 1983.
5. Herfkens, R. J., Higgins, C. B., Hricak, H., et al. Nuclear magnetic
   resonance imaging of atherosclerotic disease. *Radiology* 148:161,
   1983.

6. Hessel, S. J. Complications of Angiography and Other Catheter Procedures. In H. L. Abrams (Ed.). *Abrams Angiography: Vascular and Interventional Radiology* (3rd ed.). Boston: Little, Brown, 1983. Pp. 1041–1055.
7. Hildner, F. J., Javier, R. P., Tolentino, A., et al. Pseudo complications of cardiac catheterization: Update. *Cathet. Cardiovasc. Diagn.* 8:43, 1982.
8. Hull, R. D., Carter, C. J., Jay, R. M., et al. The diagnosis of acute, recurrent, deep-vein thrombosis: A diagnostic challenge. *Circulation* 67:901, 1983.
9. Lipchik, E. O., and Altman, D. P. Phlegmasia cerulea dolens. *Radiology* 133:81, 1979.
10. Strandness, D. E., Jr. Thrombosis detection by ultrasound, plethysmography, and phlebography. *Semin. Nucl. Med.* 7:213, 1977.
11. Williams, G. M., Harrington, D., Burdick, J., et al. Mural thrombus of the aorta: An important, frequently neglected cause of large peripheral emboli. *Ann. Surg.* 194:737, 1981.

Malignant Disease

46

Bone Metastases

Barbara J. McNeil

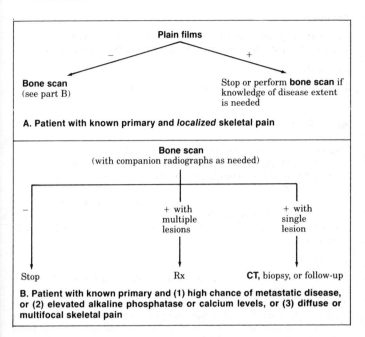

Plain films

− / +

Bone scan
(see part B)

Stop or perform **bone scan** if knowledge of disease extent is needed

A. Patient with known primary and *localized* skeletal pain

Bone scan
(with companion radiographs as needed)

− + with multiple lesions + with single lesion

Stop Rx **CT,** biopsy, or follow-up

B. Patient with known primary and (1) high chance of metastatic disease, or (2) elevated alkaline phosphatase or calcium levels, or (3) diffuse or multifocal skeletal pain

Typical Patient

Individual initially presenting with either a primary extraosseous tumor or a primary bone tumor likely to have metastasized to bone

Individual during follow-up, after treatment of intraosseous or extraosseous malignancy likely to have metastasized to bone

Typical Disorder(s)

Metastatic or primary bone tumors

Many benign processes (e.g., arthritides, osteoid osteoma, Paget's disease)

Plain Films

A simple, rapid method of screening the skeleton, which is useful with some osteolytic and with most osteoblastic lesions but is less sensitive to small lesions than radionuclide bone scans

Drawbacks

Needs 50% of cortical bone destruction for abnormalities to be visible

Sensitivity

For detecting bone metastases: lower than bone scan
For differentiating benign from malignant processes: high

Specificity

For showing normal bone as normal: high

Bone Scan

Noninvasive, generally universally available
Provides overview of abnormalities in entire skeleton
Is abnormal in areas of either new bone production or increased blood flow
Requires companion radiographs to rule out benign disease as cause of increased activity
Excellent baseline for following patients with known malignancy

Drawbacks

Even with companion radiographs, sometimes cannot distinguish benign from malignant causes of increased activity
Requires 2- to 3-hour delay from injection to imaging
In patients with breast cancer or prostate cancer on chemo- or hormonal therapy, sometimes difficult to tell progressive from healing lesions ("flare" phenomenon)
Not sensitive for multiple myeloma lesions (see below)—radiography better
Less sensitive than I^{131} scans for detecting bone metastases from carcinoma of thyroid

Comments

The presence or absence of bone pain neither rules in nor rules out bone metastases
About 75% of patients with abnormal bone scans and abnormal radiographs initially will show abnormal radiographs by 6 months
For solitary lesions with normal radiographs the probability of a metastasis varies with location: 80% for vertebral lesions and less than 15% for rib lesions
CT is useful in the evaluation of solitary lesions, particularly of the vertebrae

Sensitivity

The most sensitive examination in the search for bone metastases (except for multiple myeloma and tumors of the thy-

Table 46-1. Percent of Patients with Bone Scan Suggestive of Metastatic Disease at Time of Their Initial Presentation

Tumor	Stage I*	Stage II	Stage III
Extraosseous Tumors			
Bladder	——— 5% ———		15%
Breast	2%	2%	20%
Cervix	——— 0% ———		18%
Lung			
Asymptomatic patient	——— 8% ———		
Symptomatic patient	——— 32% ———		41%
Ovarian	——— 0% ———		8%
Prostate	5%	10%	20%
Renal cell	——— 7.5% ———		
Osseous Tumors			
Ewing's sarcoma at presentation	——— 11% ———		
Osteosarcoma at presentation	——— 3% ———		

*In general, these stages correspond to International TNM Classification. For further details, the reader should consult the original references.
Source: Data from B. J. McNeil. Value of bone scanning in neoplastic disease. *Semin. Nucl. Med.* 14:277, 1984.

roid); detects more than *98%* of untreated metastases that are detectable by any imaging method (Table 46-1)
False negatives can occur in patients with
> Multiple myeloma
> Thyroid cancer
> Any tumor that has extensive destructive component without any new bone production
> Small lytic lesions only
> Oat cell cancer

Specificity

For showing completely normal bone: high
For differentiating malignant from benign disease: only moderate because any process causing new bone production will lead to positive study
Such *false positive* causes are:
> Paget's disease
> Arthritis
> Fibrous dysplasia
> Infection
> Trauma, new or old

Additional Comments

BREAST

After initial diagnosis and therapy about 20% of patients with initially normal scans will develop bone metastases by 5–8 years [17]; few occur before 1 year

Patients with either advanced stage initially or axillary nodal involvement are more likely to convert from normal to abnormal scans in the follow-up period than those without

LUNG

A significant proportion (25%) of patients with bronchogenic carcinoma will have bone scans or radiographs indicating metastatic disease even in the presence of a normal bone marrow biopsy [13]

MULTIPLE MYELOMA

On a lesion-by-lesion basis radiographs are more sensitive than bone scans; however, few patients have a totally *normal* scan [20]

When bone scans show increased activity (instead of normal or decreased activity) associated pathological fracture is likely [3]

OSTEOSARCOMA

Patients frequently (20%) develop bone metastases before they develop lung metastases

PROSTATE

There are few if any data on the percentage of asymptomatic individuals developing abnormal bone scans after initial treatment because of the usual limitation of therapy to symptomatic patients

Abnormal alkaline or acid phosphatase levels are found in only about 50% of patients with bone metastases

Computed Tomography (CT) of Bone

Broad dynamic range permits viewing both bone and soft tissues on the same image

Combines excellent contrast resolution with good spatial resolution

Presents structures in clear cross-sectional form, free of confusion from overlapping shadows

Sometimes useful for showing benign cause of increased uptake on bone scans in patients with normal radiographs

Drawbacks

Requires companion radiographs and bone scans as well as a localizing (scoutview) device for accurate placement of slices and proper interpretation

Generally possible to examine only limited area of skeleton
Even with companion radiographs and bone scans, sometimes cannot distinguish benign from malignant lesions

Comments

Not useful as a screening tool; may clarify equivocal cases, however
May help select site for guided needle biopsy
Data on its characteristics (sensitivity and specificity) are extremely limited

Sensitivity

For detecting bone metastases no exact data: likely high, probably lower than that of bone scans
> In the calvarium results of CT and bone scans usually agree; however, each modality occasionally finds lesions not seen on the other [9]

For showing benign disease as cause of increased activity on bone scan: high
> In 20 breast cancer patients with abnormal bone scans and normal radiographs, CT confirmed metastases in 11 of 20, showed degenerative disease in 3 of 20, and was normal in 6 of 20; among the normal group there were no metastases 8 to 16 months later [12]

False negatives can occur if
> Lesions are small
> Bony changes are minimal
> Area involved is not covered by CT slices

Specificity

For showing normal bone as normal: high
False positives for detection can occur
> When technical artifacts are present
False positives for diagnosis can occur
> When benign lesions are called malignant

Contribution of Magnetic Resonance Imaging [11]

May corroborate presence of bone metastases in certain cases

References

1. Castillo, L. A., Yeh, S. D. J., Leeper, L. R., et al. Bone scans in bone metastases from functioning thyroid carcinoma. *Clin. Nucl. Med.* 5:200, 1980.
2. Citrin, D. L. The role of the bone scan in the investigation and treatment of bone cancer. *CRC Crit. Rev. Diagn. Imaging* 13:39, 1980.
3. Frank, J. W., LeBesque, S., and Buchanan, R. B. The value of bone imaging in multiple myeloma. *Eur. J. Nucl. Med.* 7:502, 1982.

4. Harbert, J. C. Efficacy of Bone and Liver Scanning in Malignant Disease. Facts and Opinions. In L. M. Freeman and H. S. Weissman (Eds.). *Nuclear Medicine Annual.* New York: Raven Press, 1982.

5. Harbert, J. C., Rocha, L., Smith, F. P., et al. The efficacy of radionuclide bone scans in the evaluation of gynecologic cancers. *Cancer* 49:1040, 1982.

6. Harbin, W. P. Metastatic disease and the nonspecific bone scan: Value of spinal computed tomography. *Radiology* 145:105, 1982.

7. Helms, C. A., Cann, C. E., Brunelle, F. O., et al. Detection of bone marrow metastases using quantitative computed tomography. *Radiology* 140:745, 1981.

8. Hooper, R. G., Beechler, C. R., and Johnson, M. C. Radioisotope scanning in initial staging of bronchogenic carcinoma. *Am. Rev. Respir. Dis.* 118:279, 1978.

9. Kido, D. K., Gould, R. Taati, F., et al. Comparative sensitivity of CT scans, radiographs and radionuclide bone scans in detecting metastatic calvarial lesions. *Radiology* 128:371, 1978.

10. McNeil, B. J. Value of bone scanning in neoplastic disease. *Semin. Nucl. Med.* 14:277, 1984.

11. Moon, K. L., Genant, H. K., Helms, C. A., et al. Musculoskeletal application of nuclear magnetic resonance. *Radiology* 147:161, 1983.

12. Muindi, J., Coombes, R. C., Golding, S., et al. The role of computed tomography in the detection of bone metastases in breast cancer patients. *Br. J. Radiol.* 56:233, 1983.

13. Ohnoshi, T., Hiraki, S., Nakata, Y., et al. Bone marrow examination for detection of metastases in patients with bronchogenic carcinoma: An evaluation of 107 patients. *Acta Med. Okayama* 36:141, 1982.

14. Paulson, D. F., and the Uro-Oncology Research Group. The impact of current staging procedures in assessing disease extent of prostatic adenocarcinoma. *J. Urol.* 121:300, 1979.

15. Pollen, J. P., Gerber, K., Washburn, W. L., et al. Nuclear bone imaging in metastatic cancer of the prostate. *Cancer* 47:2585, 1981.

16. Pollen, J. J., Witztum, K. F., and Ashburn, W. L. The flare phenomenon on radionuclide bone scan in metastatic prostate cancer. *A.J.R.* 142:773, 1984.

17. Roberts, M. M., and Hayward, J. L. Bone scanning and early breast cancer: Five year follow-up. *Lancet* 1:997, 1983.

18. Rosen, P. R., and Murphy, K. G. Bone scintigraphy in the initial staging of patients with renal cell carcinoma. *J. Nucl. Med.* 25:289, 1984.

19. Stoll, B. A., and Parbhoo, S. *Bone Metastases. Monitoring and Treatment.* New York: Raven Press, 1983.

20. Woolfenden, J. M., Pitt, M. J., Durie, B. G. M., et al. Comparison of bone scintigraphy and radiography in multiple myeloma. *Radiology* 134:723, 1980.

47

Hepatic Metastases in Nonlymphomatous Tumors

David E. Drum

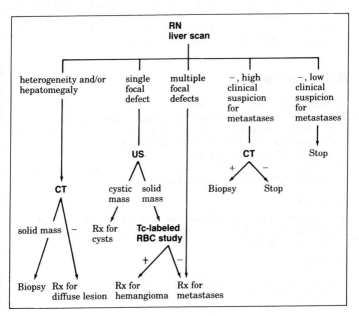

Typical Patient

Individual with known carcinoma outside the liver in whom the question of metastases is present

Individual with known metastases, on therapy, in whom the progress of the lesion is being followed

Typical Disorder(s)

Metastases from carcinomas of the lung, breast, colon and rectum, stomach and pancreas, soft tissue sarcomas, malignant melanoma, and gestational trophoblastic tumors

Comments

About 30% of patients with liver metastases will have normal liver function tests [14]

Some tumors (e.g., colorectal, gestational trophoblastic, stomach, pancreas) present with focal liver lesions, and others (e.g., breast, lung) with small diffuse lesions; the former are easier to diagnose

Sensitivities for all imaging tests are higher in more advanced metastatic disease of the liver compared to early disease

This algorithm is less useful for ovarian cancer because its metastases to the liver involve studding of Glisson's capsule and are extremely small

Hemangiomas, the most common benign tumors of the liver, are identified with great accuracy by blood pool scintigraphy with Tc-99m labeled red blood cells [6, 10]. Because of its ease and rapidity, this procedure is recommended for any solid hepatic lesion(s) of a clinically undefined nature.

Radionuclide (RN) Liver Scan

Identifies location of metastases

Indicates presence of certain other liver abnormalities

Independent of various therapeutic appliances and intra-abdominal conditions (e.g., metal clips, gas)

Rapid—less than 30 minutes

Sensitivity and specificity appear to be greater with tomographic rather than with planar imaging [2]

Drawbacks

Potential resolution relatively low: 6–8 mm in vivo at best

Liver impingement from external tumor or other processes not definitely identified

Sensitivity

Average about *87%* [1, 9, 11–14] with range of *75–95%*

False negatives can occur

    With deep-seated lesions

    With lesions beneath the limits of physical/technical resolution

    With widespread microscopic metastases

Specificity

Average about *80%* [1, 9, 11–14] with range of about *70–90%*

False positives can occur

    With incorrect interpretation of normal anatomical structures, particularly in the porta hepatis (ultrasound helpful in resolving these discrepancies)

    If focal or regional blood flow abnormalities are created by parenchymal disease

    With cysts, hemangiomas, and some cases of focal nodular hyperplasia

Comment

False positives can be reduced in patients with breast cancer if scans are interpreted as abnormal only when CEA is elevated above 1.0 ng/ml [13]

Computed Tomography (CT) of the Liver

Detects presence and location of metastases and other lesions, as well as a variety of abnormalities in adjacent organs

For some tumors (e.g., colon), this procedure is useful in determining whether a metastasis is in a surgically resectable area and whether any extrahepatic lesion would preclude a possibly curative procedure; however, with this indication (curative procedure) CT studies are falsely negative about 30% of time

Contrast enhancement heightens detection rate

Drawbacks

Radiation exposure higher than any other method to examine the liver or biliary tract

Potential allergic reaction to contrast media (about 1%)

Limited availability

Comment

In oat cell carcinoma of the lung, CT is probably the primary approach because of its ability to search for adrenal metastases at the same time; adrenal metastases may occur prior to liver metastases

Sensitivity

Averages about *90%* [1, 9, 11, 12, 14], with range of *75–96%*

False negatives can occur with

    Microscopic metastases

    Isodense metastases

    Metastases in a liver section not examined by a CT slice

Specificity

Average *87%*, with range of *85–92%* [1, 9, 11, 12, 14]

False positives can occur with

    Misinterpretation of normal structures

    Focal necrosis

    Focal benign lesions

Hepatic Ultrasound (US)

Identifies presence and location of metastases and nonmalignant lesions as well as abnormalities in adjacent structures

Rapid, inexpensive, generally available

Drawbacks

Requires skilled operator

Results may be affected by extensive abdominal gas, metal clips, drains, obesity, or ascites

Sensitivity

Averages *73%*, with wide range (*60–82%*) [1, 11, 12]
False negatives can occur from
   Microscopic disease beneath the limits of resolution
   Ultrasonically isodense macroscopic disease
   Disease foci not included in the section examined or obscured by shadows from other structures

Specificity

Averages *80%*, with wide range (*50–94%*) [1, 11, 12]
False positives can occur from
   Misinterpreting normal structures
   Focal benign disease
   Misinterpreting echogenicity at high instrument gain

Labeled Red Blood Cell (RBC) Study for Hemangioma

Identifies presence and location of hemangiomas
May help to identify hepatocellular carcinoma

Drawbacks

Moderate radiation dose to the liver (4 rads) and spleen (4 rads) from a 20-mCi administered dose
Must delay 24 hours after a radiocolloid scan

Comments

The study includes both an initial flow study (30 frames at 1.5 sec each) followed immediately and at 1–2 hours by conventional 3-view planar imaging. Single photon emission CT (SPECT) may be useful for hemangiomas near the spleen or heart blood pools.

Sensitivity

Approximately *90%* [6, 10]
False negatives can occur
   With fibrotic or thrombosed hemangiomas

Specificity

Approximately *100%* [6, 10]

Contribution of Magnetic Resonance Imaging [3, 7]

Similar to contributions of CT and ultrasound
Increment of diagnostic information gain relative to CT and ultrasound is unknown

References

1. Alderson, P. O., Adams, D. F., McNeil, B. J., et al. Computed tomography, ultrasound, and scintigraphy of the liver in patients with colon or breast carcinoma: A prospective comparison. *Radiology* 149:225, 1983.
2. Brendel, A. J., Leccia, F., Drouillard, J., et al. Single photon emission computed tomography (SPECT), planar scintigraphy, and transmission computed tomography: A comparison of accuracy in diagnosing focal hepatic disease. *Radiology* 153:527, 1984.
3. Buonocore, E., Borkowski, G. P., Pavlicek, W., et al. NMR imaging of the abdomen: Technical considerations. *AJR* 141:1171, 1983.
4. Drum, D. E. How shall we view the liver? *Postgrad. Radiol.* 2:267, 1982.
5. Drum, D. E., Detection of hepatic space-occupying lesions by nuclear medicine techniques. *Postgrad. Radiol.* 2:305, 1982.
6. Front, D., Royal, H. D., Israel, O., et al. Scintigraphy of hepatic hemangiomas: The value of Tc-99m labeled red blood cells. Concise communication. *J. Nucl. Med.* 22:684, 1981.
7. Higgins, C. B., Goldberg, H., Hricak, H., et al. Nuclear magnetic resonance imaging of vasculature of abdominal viscera: Normal and pathologic features. *AJR* 140:1217, 1983.
8. Lewis, E. Screening for diffuse and focal liver disease: The case for hepatic sonography. *J Clin Ultrasound* 12:67, 1984.
9. Miller, D. L., Rosenbaum, R. C., Sugarbaker, P. H., et al. Detection of Hepatic Metastases: Comparison of EOE-13 computed tomography and scintigraphy. *AJR* 141:931, 1983.
10. Rabinowitz, S. A., McKusick, K. A., and Strauss, H. W. ^{99m}Tc red blood cell scintigraphy in evaluating focal liver lesions. *AJR* 143:63, 1984.
11. Smith, T. J., Kemeny, M. M., Sugarbaker, P. H., et al. A prospective study of hepatic imaging in the detection of metastatic disease. *Ann. Surg.* 195:486, 1982.
12. Snow, J. H., Jr., Goldstein, H. M., and Wallace, S. Comparison of scintigraphy, sonography, and computed tomography in the evaluation of hepatic neoplasms. *Am. J. Roentgenol.* 132:915, 1979.
13. Sugarbaker, P. H., Beard, J. O., and Drum, D. E. Detection of hepatic metastases from cancer of the breast. *Am. J. Surg.* 133:531, 1977.
14. Temple, D. F., Parthasarathy, K. L., Bakshi, S. P., et al. A comparison of isotopic and computerized tomographic scanning in the diagnosis of metastasis to the liver in patients with adenocarcinoma of the colon and rectum. *Surg. Gynecol. Obstet.* 156:205, 1983.

Head and Neck Malignancies: Initial Staging

William D. Kaplan and Thomas J. Ervin

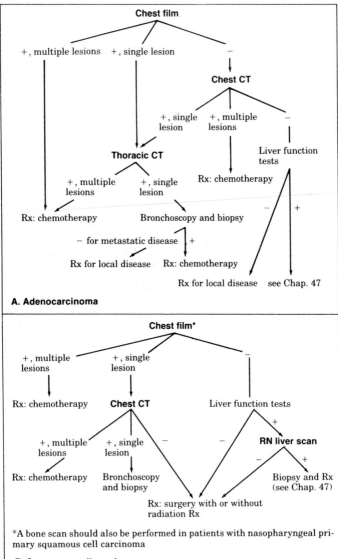

A. Adenocarcinoma

*A bone scan should also be performed in patients with nasopharyngeal primary squamous cell carcinoma

B. Squamous cell carcinoma

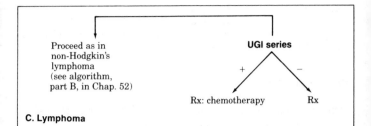

C. Lymphoma

Proceed as in non-Hodgkin's lymphoma (see algorithm, part B, in Chap. 52)

UGI series

+ Rx: chemotherapy

− Rx

Typical Patient

Individual with malignancy arising above the clavicles, usually originating from the upper aerodigestive tract

Typical Disorder(s)

Squamous cell carcinoma
Adenocarcinoma
Lymphoma
Miscellaneous malignancies
> Sarcomas, particularly embryonal or alveolar rhabdomyosarcoma arising in the sinuses or orbit
> Mucosal melanoma
> Olfactory neuroblastoma (esthesioneuroblastoma)

Comments

Types of disorder(s) being evaluated:

SQUAMOUS CELL CARCINOMA

This tumor represents 90% of the malignancies arising in the head and neck region and is associated with smoking and alcohol abuse. Stages I and II head and neck cancer have no distant metastases at presentation by definition. Stages III and IV frequently have distant spread of the disease [3, 5]; in up to 25% of patients metastases occur usually to the lung, bone, and liver—in that order.

ADENOCARCINOMA

Adenocarcinoma of salivary gland may present as a mass in the head and neck region; histological determination of aggressiveness is important in determining survival. Low-grade lesions are almost always cured with surgical resection and/or radiation therapy, with a very low incidence of distant metastases. High-grade malignancy, particularly adenoid cystic carcinoma has a 50% incidence of distant metastases as the cause of failure (lung and occasionally liver).

LYMPHOMA

Primary lymphomas of the head and neck region constitute up to 5% of what are considered extranodal non-Hodgkin's lymphomas. They often arise in the nasopharynx, faucial tonsils, and base of tongue. There is approximately a 10% incidence of gastrointestinal involvement either at the time of diagnosis or later on in the clinical course of the disease. Cervical adenopathy may be present in these cases [3].

Plain Chest Film

Compared with other radiological procedures for lung evaluation, fewer false positives are defined

Drawbacks

High false negative rate

Comment

For detecting pulmonary metastases (all cell types), a negative chest film was associated with positive findings following CT scans of the thorax or whole lung tomography (WLT) in 35% of patients (8/23) [4]

Sensitivity

For detecting metastatic nodules: low; chest films detect fewer nodules than either CT or WLT by factors of 0.3 and 0.5 respectively [6]; resolution for nodules is about 4 mm

Specificity

For showing normal lung: very high; metastatic deposits are found in 90% of resected nodules [6]

Thoracic Computed Tomography (CT)

Offers the best definition of very small metastatic deposits
Excellent for visualizing the mediastinum (but in this tumor parenchyma is more heavily involved)
Better than chest films and conventional whole lung tomography for detecting nodules, particularly pleural or subpleural

Drawbacks

Potential allergic reaction to contrast material
Does not differentiate benign from malignant processes

Sensitivity

For detecting metastatic nodules: high. In comparison to conventional tomography, in 48% of patients (patients weighted heavily towards sarcomas) CT found 59% more nodules. It detected 78% of all nodules greater than 3 mm [4].

Specificity

For showing normal lung parenchyma: moderate. Lower than that of chest radiographs and conventional whole lung tomography. Among nodules resected at surgery, only 66% are metastatic [4].

Radionuclide (RN) Liver-Spleen Scan

See Chapter 47, page 240, for detailed description

Sensitivity

Average about *87%*, with range of *75–95%*
False negatives can occur
    With deep-seated lesions
    With lesions beneath the limits of physical/technical resolution
    With widespread microscopic metastases

Specificity

Average about *80%*, with range of about *70–90%*
False positives can occur
    With incorrect interpretation of normal anatomical structures, particularly in the porta hepatis (ultrasound helpful in resolving these discrepancies)
    If focal or regional blood flow abnormalities are created by parenchymal disease
    With cysts, hemangiomas, and some cases of focal nodular hyperplasia

Upper Gastrointestinal (UGI) Series for Lymphoma

10% of patients with head and neck lymphoma will have GI involvement

Comments

Requires fasting from midnight the previous night

Sensitivity

For detecting lymphomatous involvement of stomach: moderate

Specificity

For showing normal gastric mucosa: moderate

Contribution of Magnetic Resonance Imaging [1, 9]

Neoplastic and nodal involvement can be readily differentiated from blood vessels and muscles
There is the potential for its replacing CT as the staging method of choice

References

1. Dillon, W. P., Mills, C. M., Kjos, B., et al. Magnetic resonance imaging of the nasopharynx. *Radiology* 152:731, 1984.
2. Ervin, T. J., Karp, D. D., Weichselbaum, R. R., et al. Role of chemotherapy in the multidisciplinary approach to advanced head and neck cancer: Potentials and problems. *Ann. Otol. Rhinol. Laryngol.* 90:506, 1981.
3. Evans, C. A review of non-Hodgkin's lymphomata of the head and neck. *Clin. Oncol.* 7:23, 1981.
4. Muhm, J. R., Brown, L. R., and Crowe, J. K. Use of computed tomography in the detection of pulmonary nodules. *Mayo Clin. Proc.* 52:345, 1977.
5. Probert, J. C., Thompson, R. W., and Bagshaw, M. A. Patterns of spread of distant metastases in head and neck cancer. *Cancer* 33:127, 1974.
6. Schaner, E. G., Chang, A. E., Doppman, J. L., et al. Comparison of computed and conventional whole lung tomography in detecting pulmonary nodules: A prospective radiologic-pathologic study. *AJR* 131:51, 1978.
7. Smith, T. J., Kemeny, M. M., Sugarbaker, P. H., et al. A prospective study of hepatic imaging in the detection of metastatic disease. *Ann. Surg.* 195:486, 1982.
8. Spiro, R. H., Huvos, A. G., and Strong, E. W. Adenocarcinoma of salivary origin: Clinicopathologic study of 204 patients. *Am. J. Surg.* 144:423, 1982.
9. Stark, D. D., Moss, A. A., Gamsu, G., et al. Magnetic resonance imaging of the neck. Part II: Pathologic findings. *Radiology* 150:455, 1984.

Breast Carcinoma: Initial Staging

Paul C. Stomper

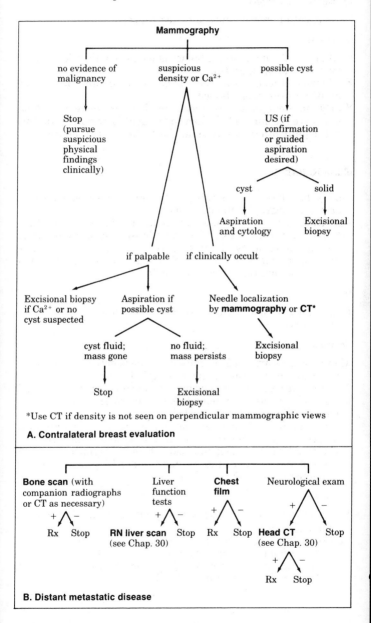

Mammography

no evidence of malignancy → **Stop** (pursue suspicious physical findings clinically)

suspicious density or Ca^{2+}

possible cyst → US (if confirmation or guided aspiration desired)
- cyst → Aspiration and cytology
- solid → Excisional biopsy

if palpable:
- Excisional biopsy if Ca^{2+} or no cyst suspected
- Aspiration if possible cyst
  - cyst fluid; mass gone → Stop
  - no fluid; mass persists → Excisional biopsy

if clinically occult:
- Needle localization by **mammography** or **CT*** → Excisional biopsy

*Use CT if density is not seen on perpendicular mammographic views

A. Contralateral breast evaluation

Bone scan (with companion radiographs or CT as necessary)
+ → Rx
− → Stop

Liver function tests
+ → **RN liver scan** (see Chap. 30)
− → Stop

Chest film
+ → Rx
− → Stop

Neurological exam
+ → **Head CT** (see Chap. 30)
  + → Rx
  − → Stop
− → Stop

B. Distant metastatic disease

This algorithm is designed to evaluate disease in the contralateral breast at presentation as well as distant metastatic disease.

Typical Patient/Disorder

Patient with newly diagnosed breast cancer

Comments

Evaluation of contralateral breast is necessary in order to look for a second primary tumor

Evaluation of ipsilateral breast is necessary in order to look for multiple sites in one breast

Yearly mammograms are recommended for follow-up. Bone scans are recommended when the patient is symptomatic, but not usually otherwise. Annual chest films discretionary

Mammography

Ideally, low-dose, small-focal-spot (0.3 mm) film-screen systems or xeroradiography should be used

Radiation dose for two-view examination is 0.1–0.8 rads if optimal equipment is used; less for film-screen technique than for xeroradiography; the risks associated with this small dose are considered less than the potential benefits from proper evaluation and treatment initially [4]

Drawbacks

Breast compression with film-screen technique will cause some discomfort

Comments

Mammograms are used initially for disease detection and later as a baseline for comparison during follow-up

The incidence of synchronous breast cancers is about 1–4% [10]

Consecutive or asynchronous breast tumors occur at a 1% annual rate for about 20 years [6]

In an annually screened population, about 45% of cancers are detected by mammography alone and between 5 and 10% are detected by physical examination alone (5% applies to women over 50 years of age; 10% to those under 50 years). The rest are detected by both modalities [1]

Sensitivity

In a population annually screened by physical examination and mammography: about *92%* [1]

False negatives can occur if

    Soft tissue masses are obscured by benign tissue

    All breast tissue is not included on image (unusual location)

    There is observer error

Specificity

For differentiating benign from malignant lesions: low [7]; only about 25% of clinically occult lesions that are suspicious on mammography for malignancy actually end up being malignant when biopsied

Mammography or Computed Tomography (CT) for Localization

If lesion can be seen on two mammographic views, mammography should be used for needle localization; with this technique it is possible to localize to within 1 cm from the lesion for excisional biopsy

If lesion cannot be seen on two perpendicular views, CT should be used for localization [5]

Localization by either technique affords smaller excisional biopsy and better cosmetic results

Bone Scan

See Chapter 46, page 234

In early clinical stage I or II disease, percentage of patients with positive bone scans is small (2%); these patients frequently present with a single abnormal area on scan. Likelihood of abnormality representing metastasis varies with location (less than 15% if single lesion in the rib end; about 80% if in vertebra)

In later clinical disease (stage III), percentage rises to 20% and disease usually multifocal

Single lesions may be studied with CT (particularly in vertebrae) and biopsied if technically feasible and desired clinically

In 20 breast cancer patients with abnormal scans and normal x-rays, CT confirmed metastases in 11 of 20, degenerative disease in 3 of 20, and was normal in 6 of 20; in the normal group, no metastases seen 8–16 months later

During the follow-up

About 20% of patients with initially normal scans will develop bone metastases by 5–8 years

Patients with advanced stage initially or axillary nodal involvement are more likely to convert from normal to abnormal scans

In as many as 27% of patients with breast cancer being treated with chemotherapy or hormonal therapy, it is difficult to distinguish progressive bone disease from healing bone lesions (see reference 9); companion radiographs showing healing or a follow-up scan indicating *decreased* activity are signs of healing

Radionuclide (RN) Liver Scan

See Chapter 47, page 240
Rarely positive in the absence of abnormal liver function tests
With normal liver function tests, less than 5% and perhaps less
than 1% of patients will have a positive liver scan

Sensitivity

Average about *87%*, with range of *75–95%*
False negatives can occur
    With deep-seated lesions
    With lesions beneath the limits of physical/technical reso-
    lution
    With widespread microscopic metastases

Specificity

Average about *80%*, with range of about *70–90%*
False positives can occur
    If normal anatomical structures, particularly in the porta
    hepatis, are incorrectly interpreted
    If focal or regional blood flow abnormalities are caused by
    parenchymal disease
    With cysts, hemangiomas, and some cases of focal nodular
    hyperplasia

Comment

False positives can be reduced if scans are interpreted as abnormal only when CEA is elevated above 1.0 ng/ml

Plain Chest Film

Approximately 6% of breast cancer patients present with lung
lesions as the initial manifestation of metastatic disease [2]
Virtually all of them are detected on plain radiographs: only 2
of 144 patients had positive plain chest tomographs and normal chest radiographs [2]
If single lesion is present, proceed as for solitary pulmonary nodule; see Chapter 26, page 130

Head Computed Tomography (CT)

See Chapter 30, page 154
Patients without neurological symptoms or signs rarely have
abnormal studies suggesting metastasis
Among symptomatic patients, the yield increases

Sensitivity

For detecting intracranial masses in general and tumors in particular: *95–98%*

False negatives can occur

> With lesions having the same attenuation value as surrounding normal brain
>
> With small lesions adjacent to the bony calvarium

Specificity

For showing normal intracranial structures or benign disease in patients suspected of malignant tumor, using contrast-enhanced scans: *97%*

For showing normal intracranial structures or benign disease in patients suspected of malignant tumor, using noncontrast scans: *93%*

False positive readings for specific diagnoses can occur

> If infarct is mistaken for tumor (or vice versa)

Contribution of Magnetic Resonance Imaging [3, 8]

Clearly distinguishes solid from cystic masses

Promising but not yet adequately defined

References

1. Baker, L. H. Breast Cancer Detection Demonstration Project: Five-year summary report. *CA* 32:194, 1982.
2. Curtis, A. M., Ravin, C. E., Collier, P. E., et al. Detection of metastatic disease from carcinoma of the breast: Limited value of full lung tomography. *AJR* 134:253, 1980.
3. El Yousef, S. J., Duchesneau, R. H., and Alfidi, R. J. Nuclear magnetic resonance imaging of the human breast. *Radiographics* 4:113, 1984.
4. Feig, S. A. Radiation risk from mammography: Is it clinically significant? *AJR* 143:469, 1984.
5. Kopans, D. B. "Early" breast cancer detection using techniques other than mammography. *AJR* 143:465, 1984.
6. McCredie, J. A., Inch, W. R., and Alderson, M. Consecutive primary carcinomas of the breast. *Cancer* 35:1472, 1975.
7. Meyer, J. E., Kopans, D. B., Stomper, P. C., et al. Occult breast abnormalities: Percutaneous preoperative needle localization. *Radiology* 150:335, 1984.
8. Ross, R. J., Thompson, J. S., Kim, K., et al. Nuclear magnetic resonance imaging and evaluation of the human breast tissue: Preliminary clinical trials. *Radiology* 143:195, 1982.
9. Rossleigh, M. A., Lovegrove, F. T. A., Reynolds, P. M., et al. The assessment of response to therapy of bone metastases in breast cancer. *Austr. N. Z. J. Med.* 14:19, 1984.
10. Sadowsky, N. Personal communication.

Bronchogenic Carcinoma: Initial Staging

Robert D. Pugatch

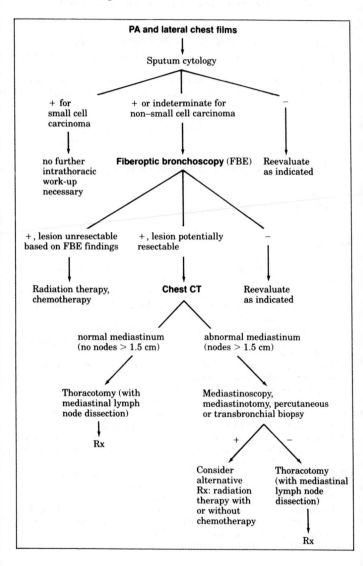

Typical Patient

Individual with signs or symptoms of bronchogenic carcinoma
Individual with tumor spreading to the mediastinum, bone, liver, brain, adrenals, or pleural/pericardial space

Typical Disorder(s)

Squamous cell carcinoma
Adenocarcinoma (including alveolar cell carcinoma)
Large cell carcinoma
Small cell carcinoma

Comments

Those patients with lung cancer presenting with a solitary pulmonary nodule are discussed in Chapter 26, p. 129
Approaches to the evaluation of patients with T2 lesions suspected of having distant disease are controversial, in large part because of a discrepancy between autopsy data, which suggest distant spread early, and radiologic data, which show a low positive yield of tests in asymptomatic patients
For example, among veterans thought to have "curable" disease, metastases for the following cell types occurred in a small sample of patients [9]:

	Epidermoid	Adenocarcinoma	Small Cell
Adrenal	5/22	7/12	4/12
Liver	5/22	2/12	7/12
Brain	2/22	5/12	2/12
Kidney	3/22	1/12	2/12

Despite these data, radionuclide liver and brain studies on asymptomatic patients thought to have operable disease are virtually never truly positive [7, 8]. Bone scans are positive about 8% of the time. Symptomatic patients have significantly higher yields of positive studies in the liver (< 10%), brain (10%), and bone (32%) [7].

Plain Chest Films (PA and Lateral)

Useful for initial detection and screening
Diagnose coexistent intrathoracic spread or other disease processes
Indicate if mediastinum is grossly abnormal, making patient possibly inoperable

Drawbacks

Mediastinal involvement may be overlooked or not evident with early lymph node metastases
Small central lesions may be nearly undetectable

Comment

The value of screening radiography remains controversial [1, 12]

Sensitivity

For central mediastinal lesions: *50%* [4]
False negatives can occur
    If nodes are too small to be visualized
    If lesion is obscured by mediastinal structures or components of the thoracic cage

Specificity

Lower than CT
False positives can occur
    If there is confusion with vascular shadows in the mediastinum or with fat deposition

Fiberoptic Bronchoscopy (FBE)

Visualizes area not seen with conventional radiographic techniques
Provides specific anatomical information and precise tissue diagnosis, especially if done with fluoroscopic guidance and appropriate aspiration, brushing, or biopsy

Drawbacks

Requires considerable expertise
Usually requires premedication (sedation)
Complications: major (e.g., laryngospasm, bronchospasm, hypoxemia, arrhythmias) in 0.08% without transbronchial biopsy, 2% with biopsy; death in .01% without biopsy, .2% with [5]
Biopsy specimens are sometimes inadequate (artifact and size)

Sensitivity

For endobronchially visible tumors when biopsy is taken: more than *90%* [5]

Specificity

High

Chest Computed Tomography (CT)

Most sensitive means for detecting mediastinal abnormality (direct spread or adenopathy)
Depicts thoracic anatomy for planning preoperative assessment

Drawbacks

Mediastinal fat or IV contrast is necessary to define mediastinum
Delivers higher radiation dose than chest radiography; equivalent to conventional tomography

May fail to differentiate contiguity from invasion of mediastinal or chest wall structures

Sensitivity

High for primary lesions 1 cm or greater in size
For nodal involvement, varies with size criteria for abnormal nodes: at 1.5 cm, sensitivity in *85–90%* range [3, 4, 6]
False negatives can occur
    With microscopic nodal involvement without enlargement

Specificity

For defining normal mediastinum, dependent on size criteria of abnormal nodes: about *80%* [3, 4, 6]
False positives can occur for nodal involvement if there is
    Reactive lymph node hyperplasia
    Previous granulomatous mediastinitis
False positives for primary lesion can occur with
    Lobar atelectasis
    Postobstructive pneumonia

Contribution of Magnetic Resonance Imaging [2, 13, 14]

There is no evidence that the contribution of MRI exceeds that of CT in staging

References

1. Boucot, K. R., and Weiss, W. Is curable lung cancer detected by semiannual screening? *JAMA* 224:1361, 1973.
2. Cohen, A. M., Creviston, S., LiPuma, J. P., et al. NMR evaluation of hilar and mediastinal lymphadenopathy. *Radiology* 148:739, 1983.
3. Daly, B. D. T., Jr., Faling, L. J., Pugatch, R. D., et al. Computed tomography: An effective technique for mediastinal staging in lung cancer. *J. Thorac. Cardiovasc. Surg.* 88:486, 1984.
4. Faling, L. J., Pugatch, R. D., Jung-Legg, Y., et al. Computed tomographic scanning of the mediastinum in the staging of bronchogenic carcinoma. *Am. Rev. Respir. Dis.* 124:690, 1981.
5. Fulkerson, W. J. Fiberoptic bronchoscopy. *N. Engl. J. Med.* 311:511, 1984.
6. Glazer, G. M., Orringer, M. B., Gross, B. H., et al. The mediastinum in non-small cell lung cancer: CT-surgical correlation. *AJR* 142:1101, 1984.
7. Hooper, R. G., Beechler, C. R., and Johnson, M. C. Radioisotope scanning in initial staging of bronchogenic carcinoma. *Am. Rev. Respir. Dis.* 118:279, 1978.
8. Kies, M. S., Baker, A. W., and Kennedy, P. S. Radionuclide scans in staging of carcinoma of the lung. *Surg. Gynecol. Obstet.* 147:175, 1978.

9. Matthews, M. J., Kanhouwa, S., Pickren, J., et al. Frequency of residual and metastatic tumor in patients undergoing curative resection for lung cancer. *Cancer Chemother. Rep.* (Part 3 [4]) 2:63, 1973.

10. Pearson, F. G., DeLarue, N. C., Ilves, R., et al. Significance of positive superior mediastinal nodes identified at mediastinoscopy in patients with resectable cancer of the lung. *J. Thorac. Cardiovasc. Surg.* 83:1, 1982.

11. Silverberg, E. Cancer statistics, 1984. *CA—A Cancer Journal for Clinicians* 34:7, 1984.

12. Stitik, F. P., and Tockman, M. S. Radiographic screening in the early detection of lung cancer. *Radiol. Clin. North Am.* 16:347, 1978.

13. Webb, W. R., Gamsu, G., Stark, D. D., et al. Magnetic resonance imaging of the normal and abnormal pulmonary hila. *Radiology* 152:89, 1984.

14. Webb, W. R., Jensen, B. G., Gamsu, G., et al. Coronal magnetic resonance imaging of the chest: Normal and abnormal. *Radiology* 153:729, 1984.

Hodgkin's Disease: Initial Staging

Maxine S. Jochelson

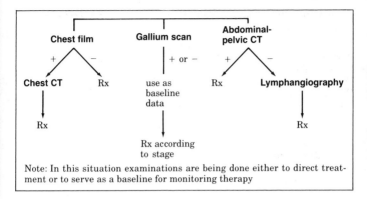

Note: In this situation examinations are being done either to direct treatment or to serve as a baseline for monitoring therapy

Typical Patient

Individual experiencing
> Lymphadenopathy with or without symptoms
> Night sweats, fever, weight loss up to 10% (B symptoms)
> Pruritus

Typical Disorder(s)

Patient with newly diagnosed Hodgkin's disease; disease with one of four histological subtypes: nodular sclerosis, mixed cellularity, lymphocyte predominant, lymphocyte depleted. Lymphocyte depleted has a worse prognosis than the other three.

Comments

Staging of this disease is according to modified Ann Arbor classification:

Stage I	Involvement of a single lymph node region or single extralymphatic organ or site
Stage II	Involvement of two or more lymph node regions on the same side of the diaphragm or localized involvement of an extralymphatic organ or site associated with a lymphocyte abnormality (II_E)
Stage III	Involvement of lymph node regions on both sides of the diaphragm This has been further broken into: III_1: Includes involvement of the upper abdominal nodes (above the celiac chain) III_2: Lower abdominal involvement
Stage IV	Diffuse or disseminated involvement of one or more extralymphatic organs with or without associated lymph node involvement

Each stage is further classified as

A   No symptoms
B   Symptoms as above

At presentation, in terms of subdiaphragmatic involvement, the following numbers hold:

	Incidence (%)
Paraaortic	34
Splenic hilar	21
Mesenteric	5
Hepatic hilar	5
Spleen	34
Liver	6

Plain Chest Film

Demonstrates mediastinal, hilar, pleural, and parenchymal involvement consistently and well

Fundamental baseline examination for following patients without thoracic disease and for monitoring effectiveness of therapy in those with thoracic disease

Drawbacks

In patients with demonstrable thoracic disease, does not show extent of disease as precisely as does CT

Comments

The role of thoracic CT has not yet been shown definitively. However, on the basis of combined data obtained in patients with Hodgkin's disease or non-Hodgkin's lymphoma, thoracic CT appears to detect a slightly greater percentage of patients with thoracic disease than do conventional radiographs. CT also defines the entire extent of disease more precisely and is therefore useful for planning of radiation therapy.

Sensitivity

For detecting mediastinal or hilar spread: no specific data for this disease; high but less so than thoracic CT

Specificity

For showing normal mediastinal and hilar structures: no specific data, but high

Computed Tomography (CT) of Thorax

Because patients with Hodgkin's disease are often treated with radiation therapy, CT is used to evaluate the extent of thoracic disease (particularly over the heart) [9] for more accurate delineation or therapy ports [16]

Sensitivity

No exact data, but higher than plain radiography

Specificity

No exact data but in mediastinum and hilum: high
No exact data but in parenchyma: moderate

Gallium Scintigraphy

Differentiates active (residual or recurrent) disease from bulky
nodal fibrosis, particularly in abdomen and mediastinum
after treatment [1]. Initial scan is necessary at time of initial
staging to see if the lymphoma is gallium-avid. If not, gallium
will not need to be repeated.
Best results obtained with high doses (7–10 mCi) and images
obtained on Anger camera rather than rectilinear scanner

Sensitivity

Highest for nodular sclerosing disease; slightly less for other cell
types—in decreasing order: lymphocyte depletion, lymphocyte
predominance, mixed cellularity [1]
For low-dose injections or images done on rectilinear scanner:
About *60%* for retroperitoneal nodes [4, 17]
About *40%* for splenic involvement [4]
About *80%* for liver involvement
With high dose and Anger camera imaging, about *90%* averaged
over all sites in one small series [1]
False negatives can occur
With small nodes or microscopic metastases
With cell types or foci that are not gallium-avid

Specificity

For low-dose injections or for images done on rectilinear scan-
ner:
About *92%* for retroperitoneal nodes [4, 17]
About *95–100%* for splenic or liver involvement [4]
Extremely high (*100%*) in one small series [1] with close clinical
and radiological correlations
False positives can occur if
GI activity is confused with tumor
Infection is confused with tumor

Abdominal Computed Tomography (CT)

Detects exact location and extent of enlarged nodes
Depicts lymph node disease in all lymph node groups if nodes
are enlarged (including parailiac, mesenteric, and retrocrural
nodal areas) as opposed to lymphangiography, which evalu-

ates only the para-aortic, common iliac, and external iliac nodes

In patients in whom recurrence is suspected, CT is the preferred initial test over lymphangiography for evaluating disease status

Drawbacks

Requires nodal enlargement for diagnosis

Possible contrast reactions—although contrast is not always required

Adequate retroperitoneal fat required for optimal visualization

Sensitivity

For detecting para-aortic nodes: average *85%* (range *77–90%*) [5, 14, 15]

For detecting splenic involvement: *50–64%* [5, 14, 15]

For detecting liver involvement: *25%* [5, 14, 15]

False negatives can occur

> If there is nodal involvement without nodal enlargement
>
> If liver and spleen involvement is diffuse and smaller than 1 cm

Specificity

For showing normal abdominal nodes: average *86%* [5, 14, 15]

False positives can occur with

> Enlarged nonneoplastic nodes
>
> Poor fat planes
>
> Unopacified bowel

For showing normal liver: moderate

For showing normal spleen: moderate, because enlarged spleens frequently occur in absence of splenic infiltration from tumor

False positives can occur

> In liver if there is a history of any liver disease, particularly alcoholic history; also if there has been recent weight loss

Lymphangiography

Indicates specific nodes for biopsy; with a KUB, shows if biopsied node was the correct one

After 1 year there is enough residual Ethiodol for adequate follow-up in 70% of patients; after 2 years this percentage drops further [7]

Drawbacks

Invasive, uncomfortable, operator dependent

Rarely, oil emboli can lead to lung infarction

Cannot evaluate nodes in hilum of liver or spleen

Rare pulmonary complications, particularly in those with prior pulmonary difficulties [8]

Sensitivity

For detecting abnormal retroperitoneal nodes: *87–93%* [4, 5, 13]
False negatives can occur with
    Microscopic disease
    Disease in nonopacified retroperitoneal nodes

Specificity

For showing normal retroperitoneal nodes: *85–92%* [4, 5, 13]
False positives can occur
    With reactive hyperplasia or fibrosis

Contribution of Magnetic Resonance Imaging [6, 11]

Demonstrates presence, size, location, and extent of lymphomatous node involvement but cannot distinguish lymphoma from metastatic lymphadenopathy
Its usefulness in locating splenic and hepatic disease is uncertain

References

1. Anderson, K. C., Leonard, R. C. F., Canellos, G. P., et al. High-dose gallium imaging in lymphoma. *Am. J. Med.* 75:327, 1983.
2. Best, J. J. K., Blackledge, G., Forbes, W. St. C., et al. Computed tomography of abdomen in staging and clinical management of lymphoma. *Br. Med. J.* 2:1675, 1978.
3. Blackledge, G., Mamtora, H., Crowther, D., et al. The role of abdominal computed tomography in lymphoma following treatment. *Br. J. Radiol.* 54:955, 1981.
4. Castellino, R. A. Imaging techniques for staging abdominal Hodgkin's disease. *Cancer Treatment Rep.* 66:697, 1982.
5. Castellino, R. A., Hoppe, R. T., Blank, N., et al. Computed tomography, lymphography, and staging laparotomy: Correlations in initial staging of Hodgkin's disease. *AJR* 143:37, 1984.
6. Dooms, G. C., Hricak, H., Crooks, L. E., et al. Magnetic resonance imaging of the lymph nodes: Comparison with CT. *Radiology* 153:719, 1984.
7. Fabian, C. E., Nudelman, E. J., and Abrams, H. L. Postlymphangiogram film as an indicator of tumor activity in lymphoma. *Invest. Radiol.* 1:386, 1966.
8. Fuchs, W. A. Technique and Complications of Lymphography. In H. L. Abrams (Ed.). *Abrams Angiography: Vascular and Interventional Radiology* (3rd ed.). Boston: Little, Brown, 1983. Pp. 1979–1986.
9. Jochelson, M. S., Balikian, J. P., Mauch, P., et al. Peri- and paracardial involvement in lymphoma: A radiographic study of 11 cases. *AJR* 140:483, 1983.
10. Kademian, M. T., and Wirtanen, G. W. Accuracy of bipedal lymphography in Hodgkin's disease. *AJR* 129:1041, 1977.

11. Lee, J. K. T., Ling, D., Heiken, J. P., et al. Magnetic resonance imaging of abdominal and pelvic lymphadenopathy. *Radiology* 153:181, 1984.

12. Magnusson, A., Hagberg, H., Hemmingsson, A., et al. Computed tomography, ultrasound and lymphography in the diagnosis of malignant lymphoma. *Acta Radiol. Diagn.* 23:29, 1982.

13. Marglin, S., and Castellino, R. Lymphographic accuracy in 632 consecutive, previously untreated cases of Hodgkin disease and non-Hodgkin lymphoma. *Radiology* 140:351, 1981.

14. Marshall, W. H., Jr., Breiman, R. S., Harell, G. S., et al. Computed tomography of abdominal paraaortic lymph node disease: Preliminary observations with a 6 second scanner. *AJR* 128:759, 1977.

15. Redman, H. C., Glatstein, E., Castellino, R. A., et al. Computed tomography as an adjunct in the staging of Hodgkin's disease and non-Hodgkin's lymphomas. *Radiology* 124:381, 1977.

16. Rostock, R. A., Giangreco, A., Wharam, M. D., et al. CT scan modification in the treatment of mediastinal Hodgkin's disease. *Cancer* 49:2267, 1982.

17. Turner, D. A., Fordham, E. W., Ali, A., et al. Gallium-67 imaging in the management of Hodgkin's disease and other malignant lymphomas. *Semin. Nucl. Med.* 8:205, 1978.

Non-Hodgkin's Lymphoma: Initial Staging

Maxine S. Jochelson

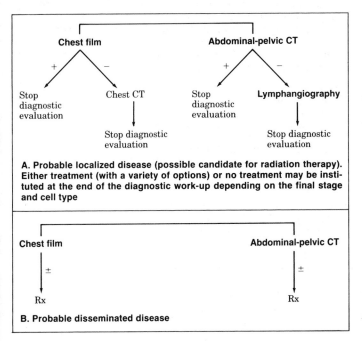

A. Probable localized disease (possible candidate for radiation therapy). Either treatment (with a variety of options) or no treatment may be instituted at the end of the diagnostic work-up depending on the final stage and cell type

B. Probable disseminated disease

Typical Patient/Disorder

Patient initially presenting with non-Hodgkin's lymphoma (NHL)

Comments

Non-Hodgkin's lymphoma refers to a broad spectrum of disease entities with differing natural histories and prognoses. Diagnostic and treatment decisions vary primarily with cell type.

Precise staging is important in prognosis, management, and follow-up. If initial treatment is unsuccessful in NHL, the salvage rate is low.

Patients with aggressive cell types generally require chemotherapy, whereas those with less aggressive cell types may not. Radiation therapy alone is reserved primarily for patients with less aggressive tumors, having stage I disease. Vigorous staging is therefore done if localized disease is suspected.

Lymph node spread is noncontiguous, and extranodal disease may be present

For patients with NHL it is essential for the radiologist to know
the pathological classification of the tumor and its natural
history so that appropriate diagnostic and treatment decisions can be made. There are at least five different pathological classifications. The Rappaport is based on the anatomy of
the pathological cell and the Lukes Collins is based on im-
munological characteristics. A "Working Formulation" has recently been devised and is shown below [4]. Low-grade lymphomas have the best prognosis.

Low Grade
A. Malignant lymphocytic
    Small lymphocytic
        Consistent with chronic lymphocytic leukemia
        Plasmacytoid
B. Malignant lymphoma, follicular
    Predominantly small cleaved cell
        Diffuse areas
        Sclerosis

Intermediate Grade
D. Malignant lymphoma, follicular
    Predominantly large cell
        Diffuse areas
        Sclerosis
E. Malignant lymphoma, diffuse
    Small cleaved cell
F. Malignant lymphoma, diffuse
    Mixed, small and large cell
        Sclerosis
        Epitheloid cell component
G. Malignant lymphoma, diffuse
    Large cell
        Cleaved cell
        Noncleaved cell
        Sclerosis

High Grade
H. Malignant lymphoma
    Large cell, immunoblastic
        Plasmacytoid
        Clear cell
        Polymorphous
        Epitheloid cell component
 I. Malignant lymphoma
    Lymphoblastic
        Convoluted cell
        Nonconvoluted cell
 J. Malignant lymphoma
    Small noncleaved cell
        Burkitt's
        Follicular areas

Monitoring of patients with NHL after initial diagnosis and evaluation depends on the pathological cell type, treatment type, and response to treatment

Plain Chest Film

Demonstrates mediastinal, hilar, pleural, and parenchymal involvement consistently and well

Fundamental baseline examination for following patients without thoracic disease and for monitoring effectiveness of therapy in those with thoracic disease

Drawbacks

In patients with demonstrable thoracic disease, does not show extent of disease as precisely as does CT; however, because of the systemic nature of therapy, this information may not be necessary

Comments

The role of thoracic CT has not yet been shown definitively. However, on the basis of combined data obtained in patients with Hodgkin's disease or non-Hodgkin's lymphoma, thoracic CT appears to detect a slightly greater percentage of patients with thoracic disease than do conventional radiographs. CT also defines the entire extent of disease more precisely and is therefore useful if planning for radiation therapy.

Sensitivity

For detecting mediastinal or hilar spread: no specific data for this disease; high but less so than thoracic CT

Specificity

For showing normal mediastinal and hilar structures: no specific data, but high

Abdominal-Pelvic Computed Tomography (CT)

Can detect lymph node disease in all lymph node groups (including retroperitoneal, mesenteric, and retrocrural nodal areas)

Can simultaneously evaluate spleen and liver but is of limited diagnostic value

Comments

Few patients with this disease go on to staging laparotomies because of the common use of systemic treatment for all but patients with stage I disease; thus, the availability of data on sensitivity and specificity is weak

Despite the above, the following estimates can be made:

For detecting para-aortic nodes: about *80–85%*

For detecting mesenteric nodes: slightly lower than for para-aortic nodes, about *75%*

For detecting splenic involvement: about *50–60%*

For detecting liver involvement: about *25%*

False negatives can occur if

> There is lymph node involvement without lymph node enlargement

> There is diffuse liver or spleen disease below resolution of instrument

For showing normal lymph nodes as normal: about *85%* [4, 8, 12]

For showing normal liver as normal: high

For showing normal spleen as normal: moderate, because enlarged spleens frequently occur in absence of splenic infiltration from tumor

False positives can occur if

> In liver if there is a history of any liver disease, particularly alcoholic history; also if recent weight loss causes fatty infiltration, or if there is incidental disease

Lymphangiography

Good for evaluating retroperitoneal lymph nodes, even those that are not enlarged

Residual contrast can help in monitoring response to therapy in follow-up period and in detecting relapse

Does not opacify mesenteric nodes, nodes in hilum of liver, spleen, or kidneys, and nodes in deep bony pelvis

Rare although serious pulmonary complications, particularly in those with prior pulmonary difficulties [7] or involvement with lymphoma

For retroperitoneal lymph nodes: *89%* [11]

False negatives can occur if

> Only microscopic metastases are present

For showing normal retroperitoneal nodes: *86%* [11]

False positives can occur

> In the presence of benign reactive changes

Contribution of Magnetic Resonance Imaging [5, 9]

Demonstrates presence, size, location, and extent of lymphomatous node involvement but cannot distinguish lymphoma from metastatic lymphadenopathy

Its usefulness in locating splenic and hepatic disease is uncertain

References

1. Best, J. J. K., Blackledge, G., Forbes, W. St. C., et al. Computed tomography of abdomen in staging and clinical management of lymphoma. *Br. Med. J.* 2:1675, 1978.
2. Blackledge, G., Mamtora, H., Crowther, D., et al. The role of abdominal computed tomography in lymphoma following treatment. *Br. J. Radiol.* 54:955, 1981.
3. Castellino, R. A. Imaging techniques for extent determinations for Hodgkin's disease and non-Hodgkin's lymphoma. 13th International Cancer Congress. Progress in Clinical and Biological Research. Vol. 1320 (Research and Treatment), Pp. 365–372. New York: Alan R. Liss, 1983.
4. Devita, V. T., Jr., and Hellman, S. Hodgkin's Disease and Non-Hodgkin's Lymphoma. In Devita, V. T., Jr., Hellman, S., and Rosenberg, S. A. (Eds.), *Cancer: Principles and Practice of Oncology.* Philadelphia: Lippincott, 1982. Chap. 35.
5. Dooms, G. C., Hricak, H., Crooks, L. E., et al. Magnetic resonance imaging of the lymph nodes: Comparison with CT. *Radiology* 153:719, 1984.
6. Ellert, J., and Kreel, L. The role of computed tomography in the initial staging and subsequent management of the lymphomas. *J. Comput. Assist. Tomogr.* 4:368, 1980.
7. Fuchs, W. A. Technique and Complications of Lymphography. In H. L. Abrams (Ed.). *Abrams Angiography: Vascular and Interventional Radiology* (3rd ed.). Boston: Little, Brown, 1983. Pp. 1979–1986.
8. Jones, S. E., Tobias, D. A., and Waldman, R. S. Computed tomographic scanning in patients with lymphoma. *Cancer* 41:480, 1978.
9. Lee, J. K. T., Ling, D., Heiken, J. P., et al. Magnetic resonance imaging of abdominal and pelvic lymphadenopathy. *Radiology* 153:181, 1984.
10. Lee, J. K. T., Stanley, R. J., Sagel, S. S., et al. Accuracy of computed tomography in detecting intraabdominal and pelvic adenopathy in lymphoma. *AJR* 131:311, 1978.
11. Marglin, S., and Castellino, R. Lymphographic accuracy in 632 consecutive, previously untreated cases of Hodgkin disease and non-Hodgkin lymphoma. *Radiology* 140:351, 1981.
12. Redman, H. C., Glatstein, E., Castellino, R. A., et al. Computed tomography as an adjunct in the staging of Hodgkin's disease and non-Hodgkin's lymphomas. *Radiology* 124:717, 1977.
13. Zelch, M. G., and Haaga, J. R. Clinical comparison of computed tomography and lymphangiography for detection of retroperitoneal lymphadenopathy. *Radiol. Clin. North Am.* 17:157, 1979.

Esophageal Carcinoma: Diagnosis and Initial Staging

William D. Kaplan and Robert J. Mayer

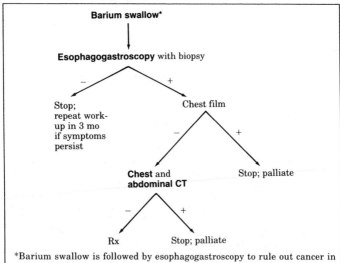

*Barium swallow is followed by esophagogastroscopy to rule out cancer in patients with a normal exam and/or to obtain tissue in abnormal exams

This algorithm is designed to rule in or rule out esophageal cancer and, if cancer is present, to stage its extent.

Typical Patient/Disorder

High risk group includes individuals with a history of excess alcohol and cigarette use, Barrett's esophagus, Plummer-Vinson syndrome, dietary deficiencies, achalasia, and concomitant head and neck cancer [1, 2]

Individuals with dysphagia, or regurgitation, or unexplained thoracic pain

Comments

Because this disease has a long asymptomatic period, extensive involvement in lymph nodes and in structures adjacent to esophagus is common

About 70% of patients with cancer of the lower third of the esophagus have abdominal lymph node involvement; more than 30% of patients with lesions of the upper third have abdominal lymph node involvement [2]

Distant metastases are most commonly found in the liver and lung [4]

During follow-up, chest radiographs should be performed annually and liver function tests or CEA titer semiannually. If either of these last two indicates liver abnormality, the liver should be reassessed using either CT or radionuclide scanning.

Barium Swallow

Demonstrates levels and extent of malignant lesion better than any other technique; length of mucosal abnormality is an important staging criterion (more than 5 cm indicates stage II) [2]

Detection of lesions provides a roadmap for endoscopist

Sensitivity

For detecting tumor of the esophagus: high. Most lesions causing symptoms are large (more than 5 mm) at presentation; a normal study usually rules out malignancy [6].

False negatives can occur
  With small mucosal lesions

Specificity

For showing a normal esophagus: high
False positives can occur
  When peptic esophagitis is confused with esophageal cancer

Endoscopy (Esophagogastroscopy) with Brushings/Biopsies

Is invariably performed when esophageal carcinoma is in question even with normal barium swallow

Comments

Successful examination is highly related to operator experience

Sensitivity

Associated brushings of tumor are usually done and are frequently more accurate for diagnosis than are biopsies; with both techniques and for tumors more than 3.5 cm in length, sensitivity for malignancy is about *90%* [4]

With smaller tumors, sensitivity drops to *60%*

Specificity

About *98%* (i.e., benign lesions of esophagus will have cytology reports read as normal 98% of time) [4]

Computed Tomography (CT) of Chest and Abdomen

Comments

Detects submucosal or extra-esophageal diseases as well as disease in adrenal glands, liver, and lymph nodes
Better for detecting direct mediastinal invasion than subdiaphragmatic spread
Sometimes used for radiation therapy planning
May underestimate length of lesion [2]; therefore the longer of two measurements (barium swallow or CT) is used for staging

Drawbacks

Cannot tell lymph node metastases if nodes are of normal size

Sensitivity

For liver metastases: about *90%* (see Chap. 47, page 241)
For detecting lymph node disease: about *75%* [2]
For detecting periesophageal lymph nodes: very low
For detecting direct mediastinal invasion; about *90%* [2]
For detecting tumor involving the aorta, pericardium, adrenal glands, and tracheobronchial tree: more than *90%* [2]
False negatives can occur
    With small nodes at any site [3]

Specificity

For all of the above areas: about *90%* [2]
False positives can occur
    For nodal involvement with inflammatory lesions, particularly common with large necrotic tumors [2]

References

1. Gilbert, H. A., and Kagan, A. R. Metastases: Incidence, Detection and Evaluation Without Histological Confirmation. In L. Weiss (Ed.). *Fundamental Aspects of Metastases.* New York: North Holland Publishing Company, 1976. Chap. 23.
2. Halvorsen, R. A., and Thompson, W. M. Computed tomographic evaluation of esophageal carcinoma. *Semin. Oncol.* 11:113, 1984.
3. Lightdale, C. J., and Winawer, S. J. Screening diagnosis and staging of esophageal cancer. *Semin. Oncol.* 11:101, 1984.
4. Rosenberg, J. C., Roth, J. A., Lichter, A. S., et al. Cancer of the Esophagus. In V. T. DeVita, S. Hellman, and S. A. Rosenberg (Eds.). *Cancer: Principles and Practice of Oncology* (2nd Ed.) Philadelphia: Lippincott, 1985. Chap. 20.
5. Schottenfeld, D. Epidemiology of cancer of the esophagus. *Semin. Oncol.* 11:92, 1984.
6. Zornoza, J., and Lindell, M. M., Jr. Radiologic evaluation of small esophageal carcinoma. *Gastrointest. Radiol.* 5:107, 1980.

Gastric Carcinoma: Diagnosis and Initial Staging

William D. Kaplan and Robert J. Mayer

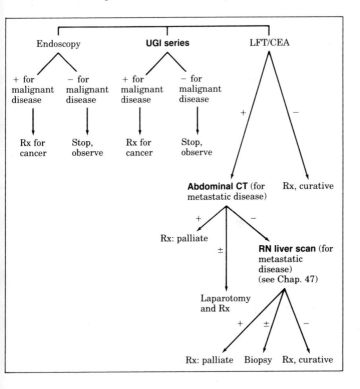

This algorithm is designed to rule in or rule out gastric cancer and, if cancer is present, to stage its extent.

Typical Patient/Disorder

Patient with symptoms of pain, early satiety, weight loss
Patient being treated for iron deficiency anemia, gastritis, gastric polyps, hiatal hernia, peptic ulcer disease, or achlorhydria
Patient with elevated serum gastrin or decreased pepsin levels
Patient with previous partial gastrectomy

Comments

At initial presentation, only about 12% of patients are free of metastases; regional disease appears in 40% and distal metastases in 36% [4]
Histologically positive nodal disease occurs in about 50% of presenting patients [4]

Liver and lung are the most common sites of distant disease—
up to 50% of patients will have liver metastases at operation
or autopsy, and up to 20% will have lung metastases [4];
spread may occur in adrenal area

Follow-up examinations usually include UGI series at 6 months
and 1 year, and annually thereafter. Liver scans are done if
patients are symptomatic, if tumor recurs, or if liver function
tests are elevated.

Upper Gastrointestinal (UGI) Series

Frequently identifies benign lesion as cause of symptoms. More-
over, nearly 100% of proven ulcers will be correctly identified
as such in these patients [7].

Monitoring presumed benign lesions during treatment is essential to decrease errors in classifying benign vs. malignant

Sensitivity

For detecting gastric cancer: between *70 and 95%* [6, 7]
False negatives can occur
    With superficial or early infiltrating disease

Specificity

For showing normal gastric mucosa: high
False positives for diagnosis can occur in inflammatory disease

Abdominal Computed Tomography (CT)

Comments

Defines disease in regional lymph nodes in the peritoneum; between 40 and 70% of patients have disease in these areas depending upon histological type and size of lesion [1, 6]

Identifies direct invasion of adjacent organs (spleen in 4%, pancreas in 15%) as well as metastatic disease (e.g., liver in 40%,
adrenal in 5%, kidneys in 5%) [5, 6]

Results of CT correlate well with findings at surgery [5]

In detecting *early* liver metastases, radionuclide studies, which
show evidence of diffuse disease, provide better results

Radionuclide (RN) Liver Scans

See Chapter 47, page 240

Comments

Early metastatic disease is frequently manifested by heteroge-
neity of uptake resulting from tumor infiltration along the
sinusoids; there is usually no derangement of hepatic architecture [2, 8]. Therefore, radionuclide studies are done even if
CT is normal.

About 40% of patients have liver metastases at presentation [6]; virtually all of these have abnormal liver function tests because of the infiltrative nature of the metastases

Sensitivity

Average about *87%,* with range of *75–95%*
False negatives can occur
> With deep-seated lesions
> With lesions beneath the limits of physical/technical resolution
> With localized microscopic metastases

Specificity

Average about *80%,* with range of about *70–90%*
False positives can occur
> With incorrect interpretation of normal anatomical structures, particularly in the porta hepatis (ultrasound is helpful in resolving these discrepancies)
> If focal or regional blood flow abnormalities are created by parenchymal disease
> With cysts, hemangiomas, and some cases of focal nodular hyperplasia

References

1. Cady, B., Ramsden, D. A., Stein, A., et al. Gastric cancer: Contemporary aspects. *Am. J. Surg.* 133:423, 1977.
2. Conn, H. O., and Yesner, R. A reevaluation of needle biopsy in the diagnosis of metastatic cancer of the liver. *Ann. Intern. Med.* 59:53, 1963.
3. Lawrence, W. T., and Lawrence, W., Jr. Gastric cancer: The surgeon's viewpoint. *Semin. Oncol* 7:400, 1980.
4. MacDonald, J. S., Gunderson, L. L., and Cohn, I., Cancer of the Stomach. In V. T. DeVita, Jr., S. Hellman, and S. A. Rosenberg (Eds.). *Cancer: Principles and Practice of Oncology.* (2nd ed.) Philadelphia: Lippincott, 1985. Chap. 21.
5. Moss, A. A., Schnyder, P., Marks, W., et al. Gastric adenocarcinoma: A comparison of the accuracy and economics of staging by computed tomography and surgery. *Gastroenterology* 80:45, 1981.
6. Olearchyk, A. S. Gastric carcinoma: A critical review of 243 cases. *Am. J. Gastroenterol.* 70:25, 1978.
7. Schulman, A., and Simpkins, K. C. The accuracy of radiological diagnosis of benign, primarily and secondarily malignant gastric ulcers and their correlation with three simplified radiological types. *Clin. Radiol.* 26:317, 1975.
8. Watson, A. J. Diffuse intra-sinusoidal metastatic carcinoma of the liver. *J. Pathol. Bacteriol.* 69:207, 1955.

Colon Carcinoma: Initial Staging

William D. Kaplan and Robert J. Mayer

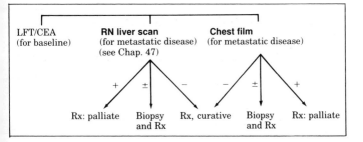

Typical Patient/Disorder

Patient in whom colon cancer has been diagnosed by barium enema, colonoscopy, sigmoidoscopy

Comments

Although surgery is performed on all patients with this disease, the presence of metastatic disease usually leads to palliative rather than curative surgery

As it spreads, the disease tends to penetrate perpendicularly through the bowel wall, with associated regional lymph node involvement

Distant metastases are most common in liver; spread to other sites occurs less often, overall less than 5% of time [4, 5]

Some patients with solitary pulmonary or hepatic metastases may be cured after resection of metastases. In liver, in particular, tests are used, therefore, to diagnose and to indicate surgical resectability (see Chap. 47 algorithm, page 239).

Elevated preoperative CEA levels are correlated with recurrence rates [9] and hence are usually done as baseline

Follow-up examination should be every 6 months for 2 years, afterwards every year, and include LFT and CEA, chest film, and colonoscopy

Radionuclide (RN) Liver-Spleen Scan

See Chapter 47, page 240

Comments

Between 15 and 25% of patients presenting with colon cancer have liver metastases; metastases from colon cancer tend to be multiple and focal, involving the deep and superficial parenchyma

CT is considered slightly more sensitive than RN scanning for detecting liver metastases, but the focal nature of lesions diminishes the difference in sensitivity between the two techniques [1]

If information regarding extrahepatic abnormalities is considered critical at the time of initial staging, the RN study should be replaced by CT; information on extrahepatic involvement is seen in about 13% of patients [1]

Sensitivity

Average about *87%,* with range of *75–95%*
False negatives can occur
  With deep-seated lesions
  With lesions beneath the limits of physical/technical resolution
  With widespread microscopic metastases

Specificity

Average about *80%,* with range of about *70–90%*
False positives can occur
  With incorrect interpretation of normal anatomical structures, particularly in the porta hepatis (ultrasound is helpful in resolving these discrepancies)
  If focal or regional blood flow abnormalities are created by parenchymal disease
  With cysts, hemangiomas, and some cases of focal nodular hyperplasia

Plain Chest Film

Comments

Only a small percentage of patients (less than 5%) present with lung metastases; in the course of their disease, between 20 and 30% of patients with colon cancer will develop lung metastases [4, 5] and hence a baseline film is advisable

In colon cancer patients with a solitary pulmonary nodule, there is a 50% chance that the nodule represents malignant disease [2]; when discovered, CT of the chest should follow (see Chap. 26, p. 129) to search for additional nodules

References

1. Alderson, P. O., Adams, D. F., McNeil, B. J., et al. Computed tomography, ultrasound and scintigraphy of the liver in patients with colon or breast carcinoma: A prospective comparison. *Radiology* 149:225, 1983.
2. Cahan, W. G., Castro, E. B., and Hajdu, S. I. The significance of a solitary lung shadow in patients with colon carcinoma. *Cancer* 33:414, 1974.
3. Drum, D. E., and Beard, J. M. Scintigraphic criteria for hepatic metastases from cancer of the colon and breast. *J. Nucl. Med.* 17:677, 1976.

4. Gilbert, H. A., and Kagan, A. R. Metastases: Incidence, Detection and Evaluation Without Histological Confirmation. In L. Weiss (Ed.). *Fundamental Aspects of Metastases.* New York: North Holland Publishing Company, 1976. Chap. 23.

5. Hoth, D. F., and Petrucci, P. E. Natural history and staging of colon cancer. *Semin. Oncol.* 3:331, 1976.

6. Knopf, D. R., Torres, W. E., Fajman, W. J., et al. Liver lesions: Comparative accuracy of scintigraphy and computed tomography. *AJR* 138:623, 1982.

7. Muhm, J. R., Brown, L. R., and Crowe, J. K. Use of computed tomography in the detection of pulmonary nodules. *Mayo Clin. Proc.* 52:345, 1977.

8. Temple, D. F., Parthasarathy, K. L., Bakshi, S. P., et al. A comparison of isotopic and computerized tomographic scanning in the diagnosis of metastasis to the liver in patients with adenocarcinoma of the colon and rectum. *Surg. Gynecol. Obstet.* 156:205, 1983.

9. Sugarbaker, P. H., Gunderson, L. L., and Wittes, R. E. Colorectal Cancer. In V. T. Devita, S. Hellman, and S. A. Rosenberg (Eds.). *Cancer: Principles and Practice of Oncology* (2nd ed.). Philadelphia: Lippincott, 1985. Chap. 25.

10. Woolley, P. V., III. Clinical manifestations of cancer of the colon and rectum. *Semin. Oncol.* 3:373, 1976.

Pancreatic Carcinoma: Initial Staging

William D. Kaplan and Robert J. Mayer

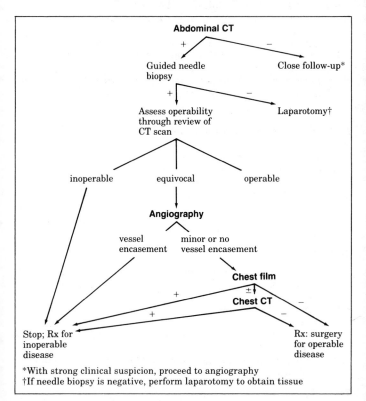

*With strong clinical suspicion, proceed to angiography
†If needle biopsy is negative, perform laparotomy to obtain tissue

Typical Patient

Individuals in whom the diagnosis of pancreatic carcinoma is strongly suspected as well as those in whom the diagnosis has already been made. In the latter group staging information is obtained.

Comments

Although some studies indicate that the sensitivity of ultrasound may be close to that of CT, other studies do not. One prospective study, for example, shows a sensitivity value of ultrasound of only 60% [8]. Hence, the algorithm begins with computed tomography.

At the time of diagnosis, about 85% of patients will already have distant or regional metastases [5]

At autopsy
Sites of direct extension of tumor vary with tumor location initially, but on average they are highest in duodenum, stomach, and less often in spleen and adrenal
Lymph nodes most commonly involved are peripancreatic (42%) and aortic or mesenteric (27%) [12]
Distant metastases are seen most commonly in the liver (62%) lung (40%) intestines (25%), and adrenal (24%) [12]
During the follow-up period these examinations are routinely done: CEA every 3 months and CT postoperatively to serve as a baseline; chest radiography is performed yearly

Abdominal Computed Tomography (CT)

Useful for identifying a wide variety of diseases in the pancreas; frequently helpful in determining whether they are benign or malignant
Visualizes the extent of disease (e.g., involvement of lymph nodes or fascial planes) and surrounding structures
Can be combined with needle biopsy for initial diagnosis of tumor (sensitivity of 76–87%) [1]

Drawbacks

Oral contrast agents are frequently necessary to distinguish bowel (which may be closely applied to pancreas) from pancreatic masses
Intravenous contrast agents are frequently needed to study potentially inflammatory lesions
Differentiating benign from malignant processes is not always possible
Minor complications (pneumothorax, syncope) occasionally occur (6%) from CT-guided biopsies [3]

Sensitivity

For detecting disease of any sort in the pancreas: nearly *90%* (range, *79–94%*) [4, 5, 8]
For detecting disease and correctly classifying it as benign or malignant: about *78%* [8]
For detecting hepatic metastases: 90% (see Chap. 47, p. 241)
Only preliminary data are available for correctly predicting resectable lesions, but possibly close to that of arteriography [9]

Specificity

For showing totally normal pancreas as normal: up to *90%* [8], with values as low as *64%* reported [5]
For showing normal liver: *87%* (see Chap. 47, p. 241)

Arteriography

Sometimes useful for differentiating benign from malignant diseases

Arterial narrowing and/or encasement suggest invasion of vessels by tumor; however, patients with tumor limited to intrapancreatic arteries and with minor vessel encasement are usually believed to have resectable disease

Encasement of hepatic or cystic arteries is a frequent sign of hepatic or gallbladder involvement

Provides a road map for the surgeon if tumor is believed to be locally resectable

Drawbacks

Complications: contrast reaction and/or secondary renal failure, rare; vascular injury and thrombosis, serious, about 1%; local hemorrhage or hematoma, nonfatal serious reactions, less than 2%; fatalities, .03% [7]

Inflammatory disease can produce vessel changes that simulate encasement

Sensitivity

For detecting cancer of the pancreas: *60–69%* [4, 5]

For differentiating pancreatic carcinoma from non-neoplastic diseases (e.g., chronic pancreatitis or pseudocyst): low [11]

For predicting resectable lesions: variable, from *43%* [17] to *72%* [16]

Specificity

For showing normal pancreas or pancreas with benign disease: *85–95%* [4, 5]

Plain Chest Film

No data exist on the percentage of individuals with lung metastases at presentation. However, the percentage at autopsy is high: 30% for carcinoma of the pancreatic head, 14% for carcinoma of the body or tail [14]. Therefore, baseline chest radiographs are routinely done.

References

1. Beazley, R. M. Percutaneous needle biopsy for diagnosis of pancreatic cancer. *Semin. Oncol.* 6:344, 1979.
2. Berg, J. W., and Connelly, R. R. Updating the epidemiologic data on pancreatic cancer. *Semin. Oncol.* 6:275, 1979.
3. Ferrucci, J. T., Jr., and Wittenberg, J. CT biopsy of abdominal tumors: Aids for lesion localization. *Radiology* 129:739, 1978.
4. Fitzgerald, P. J., Fortner, J. G., Watson, R. C., et al. The value of diagnostic aids in detecting pancreas cancer. *Cancer* 41:868, 1978.

5. Go, V. L. W., Taylor, W. F., and DiMagno, E. P. Efforts at early diagnosis of pancreatic cancer: The Mayo Clinic experience. *Cancer* 47:1698, 1981.

6. Haaga, J. R., and Alfidi, R. J. Precise biopsy localization by computed tomography. *Radiology* 118:603, 1976.

7. Hessel, S. J. Complications of Angiography and Other Catheter Procedures. In H. L. Abrams (Ed.). *Abrams Angiography: Vascular and Interventional Radiology* (3rd ed.). Boston: Little, Brown, 1983. Pp. 1041–1055.

8. Hessel, S. J., Siegelman, S. S., McNeil, B. J., et al. A prospective evaluation of computed tomography and ultrasound of the pancreas. *Radiology* 143:129, 1982.

9. Jafri, S. Z. H., Aisen, A. M., Glazer, G. M., et al. Comparison of CT and angiography in assessing resectability of pancreatic carcinoma. *AJR* 142:525, 1984.

10. Kamin, P. D., Bernardino, M. E., Wallace, S., et al. Comparison of ultrasound and computed tomography in the detection of pancreatic malignancy. *Cancer* 46:2410, 1980.

11. Levin, D. C., Wilson, R., and Abrams, H. L. The changing role of pancreatic arteriography in the era of computed tomography. *Radiology* 136:245, 1980.

12. Lisa, J. R., Trinidad, S., and Rosenblatt, M. B. Pulmonary manifestations of carcinoma of the pancreas. *Cancer* 17:395, 1964.

13. Rosch, J., Keller, F. S., and Bilbao, M. K. Radiologic diagnosis of pancreatic cancer. *Semin. Oncol.* 6:318, 1979.

14. Sindelar, W. F., Kinsella, T. J., and Mayer, R. J. Cancer of the Pancreas. In V. T. DeVita, S. Hellman, and S. A. Rosenberg (Eds.). *Cancer: Principles and Practice of Oncology* (2nd ed.). Philadelphia: Lippincott, 1985. Chap. 22.

15. Smith, E. H., Bartrum, R. J., Jr., Chang, Y. C., et al. Percutaneous aspiration biopsy of the pancreas under ultrasonic guidance. *N. Engl. J. Med.* 292:825, 1975.

16. Suzuki, T., Kawabe, K., and Imamura, M. Survival of patients with cancer of the pancreas in relation to findings on arteriography. *Ann. Surg.* 176:37, 1972.

17. Tylen, U., and Arnesjo, B. Resectability and prognosis of carcinoma of the pancreas evaluated by angiography. *Scand. J. Gastroenterol.* 8:691, 1973.

Prostatic Carcinoma: Initial Staging

Roger A. Styles and Steven E. Seltzer

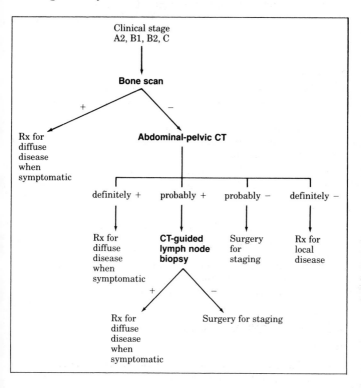

Typical Patient/Disorder

This algorithm applies to a patient in whom prostatic cancer has already been diagnosed, either incidentally in tissue removed for treatment of benign prostatic hypertrophy (stages A1 or A2) or because of symptoms or signs reflective of prostatic disease (e.g., urinary tract obstruction). This algorithm also concerns staging of those with clinical disease stages A2, B, or C. Patients with stage A1 disease require no further work-up; patients with stage D disease at presentation require only a baseline bone scan.

For this discussion the stages are defined as follows:

Stage A Tumor discovered incidentally in tissue removed for treatment of benign prostatic hypertrophy
    A1 Small focal involvement of one lobe
    A2 Multifocal or diffuse carcinoma

Stage B	Palpable carcinoma confined to prostate on digital rectal examination
	B1 Solitary nodule less than 1.5 cm
	B2 Diffuse involvement of both lobes
Stage C	Tumor extending through the prostatic capsule but has not metastasized
Stage D	Metastases, usually to bone and/or pelvic lymph nodes

Comments

At presentation the organ with the highest incidence of distant non-nodal occult metastatic disease is bone (see Chap. 46, page 233)

Locally tumor extends via the obturator, hypogastric, external iliac, and presacral lymphatics. By stage, involvement of these nodal areas is:

A2	Poorly differentiated cell type	25%
B1	Well-differentiated cell type	8–21%
B2	Moderately to poorly differentiated	14–45%
C	All cell types	40–80%

The probability of nodal involvement increases as the serum acid phosphatase value increases [6]; acid phosphatase levels also serve as baseline values

Follow-up radionuclide bone scan and acid phosphatase determinations are done annually in asymptomatic patients and at any time patient develops symptoms

Radionuclide (RN) Bone Scan

Comments

The incidence of bone scans positive for metastases ranges from 5% for stage B disease to nearly 20% for stage C disease (see Chap. 46, page 234)

During initial staging both the acid and alkaline phosphatase assays provide an insensitive (less than 50%) indicator of metastatic disease [10], although a high acid phosphatase level frequently implies bone metastases

In the follow-up evaluations of patients with stage D disease under treatment with chemo- or hormonal therapy, it is sometimes difficult to distinguish new bone disease from healing bone metastases (flare phenomenon) [4]. This occurs in 6% of patients [7].

Sensitivity

Among all patients with bone metastases, the highest of all modalities; for example, plain bone radiographs will detect disease in only two-thirds as many patients, and acid and alkaline phosphatase assays in only half as many patients [10]

Specificity

No specific data but false positive diagnoses are probably less frequent with prostatic cancer than with several other tumors (e.g., breast cancer) because of the usual multifocal nature of involvement. However, such errors can be made in the presence of Paget's disease.

Computed Tomography (CT) of Pelvis and Retroperitoneum

Identifies and localizes lymph node involvement for staging and treatment planning; examinations are sometimes equivocal, however. "Probably positive examinations" occur with one or two enlarged nodes; "probably negative" examinations occur with multiple small nodes.

Assesses size of prostate for radiotherapy, particularly for patients with stage C disease

May identify extracapsular tumor extension

Provides a good demonstration of pelvic and retroperitoneal cross-sectional anatomy

Sensitivity

For detecting lymph metastases: about *82%* [5, 12]. This considers all nodes 1.5 cm or greater as abnormal except for deep pelvic nodes (hypogastric or obturator), which are considered abnormal if greater than 1.2 cm.

False negatives for lymph node involvement can occur
    With micrometastases
    In nodes that fail to enlarge

For detecting extracapsular extension: about *32%* [2, 3]. Extracapsular extension is defined as interruption in normal contour of prostate, asymmetric enlargement of prostate, or haziness of periprostatic tissue planes

False negatives for extracapsular extension can occur
    With invasion of seminal vesicles or periprostatic fat below the threshold of detection

Specificity

For showing normal lymph nodes: *82%* [5, 12]

False positives can occur from
    Bowel loops
    Vessels
    Large benign lymph nodes

For showing normal prostatic gland: *90%* [2, 3]

False positives can occur with
    Acute or chronic inflammation
    Scar tissue from prior surgery
    Radiation fibrosis (likely only if an earlier pelvic malignancy was present)

CT-Guided Lymph Node Biopsy

Confirms stage D disease when CT interpretation is equivocal and when a suspicious lymph node is accessible to a percutaneous approach; if positive cytology is obtained, staging surgery can be avoided
Requires fine needle (22 gauge)
Can be used on an outpatient basis; requires only local anesthesia and minimal discomfort is involved

Drawbacks

Small risk of infection, bleeding

Sensitivity

No data available, but negative aspiration biopsy does not rule out nodal involvement

Specificity

No data available, but likely high

Contribution of Magnetic Resonance Imaging [1, 8]

May detect small malignant nodules within the prostate
May ultimately distinguish benign prostatic hypertrophy from malignancy
Delineates extension of neoplasm beyond the limits of the gland

References

1. Buonocore, E., Hesemann, C., Pavlicek, W., et al. Clinical and in vitro magnetic resonance imaging of prostatic carcinoma. *AJR* 143:1267, 1984.
2. Denkhaus, H., Dierkopf, W., Grabbe, E., et al. Comparative study of suprapubic sonography and computed tomography for staging of prostatic carcinoma. *Urol. Radiol.* 5:1, 1983.
3. Golimbu, M., Morales, P., Al-Askari, S., et al. CAT scanning in staging of prostatic cancer. *Urology* 18:305, 1981.
4. Levenson, R. M., Sauerbrunn, B. J., Bates, H. R., et al. Comparative value of bone scintigraphy and radiography in monitoring tumor response in systemically treated prostatic carcinoma. *Radiology* 146:513, 1984.
5. Levine, M. S., Arger, P. H., Coleman, B. G., et al. Detecting lymphatic metastases from prostatic carcinoma. Superiority of CT. *AJR* 137:207, 1981.
6. Paulson, D. F., and Uro-oncology Research Group. The impact of current staging procedures in assessing disease extent of prostatic adenocarcinoma. *J. Urol.* 121:300, 1979.
7. Pollen, J. J., Witztum, K. F., and Ashburn, W. L. The flare phenomenon on radionuclide bone scan in metastatic prostate cancer. *AJR* 142:773, 1984.

8. Poon, P. Y., McCallum, R. W., Henkelman, M. M., et al. Magnetic resonance imaging of the prostate. *Radiology* 154:143, 1985.
9. Schaffer, D. L., and Pendergrass, H. P. Comparison of enzyme, clinical, radiographic, and radionuclide methods of detecting bone metastases from carcinoma of the prostate. *Radiology* 121:431, 1976.
10. Shafer, R. B., and Reinke, D. B. Contribution of the bone scan, serum acid and alkaline phosphatase, and the radiographic bone survey to the management of newly-diagnosed carcinoma of the prostate. *Clin. Nucl. Med.* 2:200, 1977.
11. Walsh, J. W., Amendola, M. A., Konerding, K. F., et al. Computed tomographic detection of pelvic and inguinal lymph-node metastases from primary and recurrent pelvic malignant disease. *Radiology* 137:157, 1980.
12. Weinerman, P. M., Arger, P. H., Coleman, B. G., et al. Pelvic adenopathy from bladder and prostate carcinoma. *AJR* 140:95, 1983.

Testicular Carcinoma: Initial Staging

William D. Kaplan

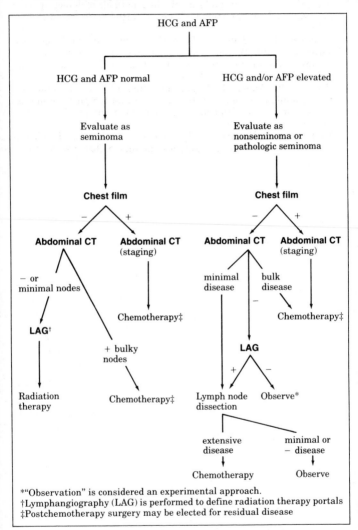

*"Observation" is considered an experimental approach.
†Lymphangiography (LAG) is performed to define radiation therapy portals
‡Postchemotherapy surgery may be elected for residual disease

Typical Patient/Disorder

Individual with a scrotal mass proven to be a malignant primary

Comments

If a tumor is called a seminoma by pathology but either or both of the tumor markers (HCG or AFP) is elevated, then the tumor is considered a pathologic seminoma; but the evaluation proceeds as shown on the left and is identical to that on non-seminoma

Even in early stage disease (stage A) 10% of patients with seminomas will have lymph node involvement [3]; in nonseminomatous tumors the percentage is higher

Surgery is curative in a large percentage of cases (90% of clinical stage A, 70–80% of stages B and C) [3]

HCG or AFP levels are elevated in more than 90% of patients with nonseminomatous tumors at presentation [3]

Recurrences correlate with elevation of HCG or AFP in 60–70% of patients [3]

Relapses occur locally and distally in lung [3]

During follow-up, HCG and AFP are done every 2 months for patients with nonseminomatous lesions; for all patients chest radiographs are done at 2-month intervals in year one and at 3- to 6-month intervals thereafter

Plain Chest Films

Excellent screening procedure for gross pulmonary metastases
Important baseline procedure for follow-up

Drawbacks

Greater false negative ratio obtained in comparison with other radiographic examinations

Sensitivity

Absolute value impossible to obtain

In relation to CT as an endpoint: 1 of 120 patients with testicular cancer had a positive thoracic CT and normal chest radiograph [5]

Comment

The above data apply to testicular cancer; other studies [7] have compared chest films to CT and whole lung tomography in various tumors and have found, on average, that 35% of patients with normal chest films will have abnormal CT or conventional whole lung tomograms

Specificity

No data available, but likely high

Abdominal Computed Tomography (CT)

Provides excellent resolution of cross-sectional anatomy and clear demonstration of tumor margins

Provides clear demonstration of nodes when enlarged

Occasionally useful for detecting simultaneous liver metastases [10]

Drawbacks

Possible contrast reactions

Requires enlarged lymph nodes and fails to detect involved nodes of normal size

Sensitivity

For retroperitoneal nodes, average of *72%,* range *65–90%* [1, 8, 10]

False negatives can occur with

    Microscopic disease

    Macroscopic disease without nodal enlargement

    Insufficient retroperitoneal fat for contrast

Comment

False negative studies pose little or no problem since all patients with minimal disease are treated in the same manner

Specificity

Greater than 90% in retroperitoneal area [1, 8, 10]

False positives can occur

    In the presence of adenopathy secondary to inflammation or fibrosis

    With misinterpretation of normal structures

Lymphangiography (LAG)

Delineates portals for radiation therapy

Demonstrates morphology of pelvic and retroperitoneal lymph nodes

Drawbacks

Invasive

Reactions to oily contrast agents 1 in 10,000

Should be avoided when possible in the presence of compromised pulmonary function

Serious pulmonary complications: 0.5%, particularly in those with prior pulmonary difficulties [2]

Contrast may lead to surrounding fibrosis, making lymph node dissection difficult; thus lymphangiography is rarely performed in patients with nonseminomatous tumors [8]

Sensitivity

For detecting nodes in retroperitoneal area: average 75% [1, 10]
False negatives can occur
> With microscopic disease
> With macroscopic disease without nodal enlargement
> From nonopacification due to either normal anatomical by-
> passing of involved nodes or postoperative alteration of
> pathways

Specificity

Varies markedly with criterion for abnormality: average about
90% (if only defects of at least 5.0 mm are considered abnormal) [1, 10]
False positives can occur
> Secondary to inflammatory changes

Contribution of Magnetic Resonance Imaging [6]

Defines tumor clearly in primary site and abnormal lymph
nodes in pelvis and retroperitoneum

References

1. Dunnick, N. R., and Javadpour, N. Value of CT and lymphography: Distinguishing retroperitoneal metastases from non-semi-
   nomatous testicular tumors. *AJR* 136:1093, 1981.
2. Fuchs, W. A. Technique and Complications of Lymphography. In
   H. L. Abrams (Ed.). *Abrams Angiography: Vascular and Interventional Radiology* (3rd ed.). Boston: Little, Brown, 1983. Pp. 1979–
   1986.
3. Garnick, M. B., Prout, G. R., and Canellos, G. P. Germinal Tumors
   of the Testis. In J. F. Holland and E. Frei III (Eds.). *Cancer Medicine* (2nd ed.). Philadelphia: Lea & Febiger, 1982. Pp. 1937–1956.
4. Hessel, S. J. Complications of Angiography and Other Catheter
   Procedures. In H. L. Abrams (Ed.). *Abrams Angiography: Vascular
   and Interventional Radiology* (3rd ed.). Boston: Little, Brown,
   1983. Pp. 1041–1055.
5. Jochelson, M. S., Garnick, M. B., Balikian, J. P., et al. The efficacy
   of routine whole lung tomography in germ cell tumors. *Cancer*
   54:1007, 1984.
6. Lee, J. K. T., Ling, D., Heiken, J. P., et al. Magnetic resonance
   imaging of abdominal and pelvic lymphadenopathy. *Radiology*
   153:181, 1984.
7. Muhm, J. R., Brown, L. R., and Crowe, J. K. Use of computed tomography in the detection of pulmonary nodules. *Mayo Clin. Proc.*
   52:345, 1977.
8. Richie, J. P., Garnick, M. B., and Finberg, H. Computerized tomography: How accurate for abdominal staging of testis tumors? *J.
   Urol.* 127:715, 1982.

9. Shehadi, W. H. Adverse reactions to intravascularly administered contrast media: A comprehensive study based on a prospective survey. *AJR* 124:145, 1975.
10. Thomas, J. L., Bernardino, M. E., and Bracken, R. B. Staging of testicular carcinoma: Comparison of CT and lymphangiography. *AJR* 137:991, 1981.

Ovarian Carcinoma: Diagnosis and Initial Staging

William D. Kaplan and Ross S. Berkowitz

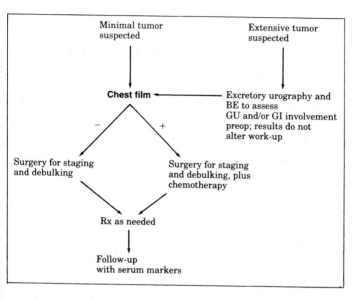

Typical Patient/Disorder

Individual presenting with pelvic mass, pelvic pain, or ascites (distention), or with a positive bimanual gynecological examination [11]

Comments

This tumor is *always* surgically staged to identify the primary site, determine the pattern of spread, and obtain tissue for tumor typing and grading [4]

Initial spread is often nodal; distant disease to lung or liver occurs less than 5% of time at initial presentation and less than 15% of time at autopsy [6]

Plain Chest Film

Virtually never positive in stage I or II disease

Positive in about 14% of patients with stage III or IV disease; this rate is not appreciably increased by computed whole lung tomography [8] since the most common finding is pleural effusion not parenchymal nodules

Contribution of Magnetic Resonance Imaging [2, 3, 5]

Excellent for demonstrating ovarian anatomy, tumor size, and extent

References

1. Amendola, M. A., Walsh, J. W., Amendola, B. E., et al. Computed tomography in the evaluation of carcinoma of the ovary. *J. Comput. Assist. Tomogr.* 5:179, 1981.
2. Bies, J. R., Ellis, J. H., Kopecky, K. K., et al. Assessment of primary gynecologic malignancies: Comparison of 0.15 T resistive MRI with CT. *AJR* 143:1249, 1984.
3. Bryan, P. J., Butler, H. E., LiPuma, J. P., et al. NMR scanning of the pelvis: Initial experience with a 0.3 T system. *AJR* 141:1111, 1983.
4. Buchsbaum, H. J., and Lifshitz, S. Staging and surgical evaluation of ovarian cancer. *Semin. Oncol.* 11:227, 1984.
5. Butler, H., Bryan, P. J., LiPuma, J. P., et al. Magnetic resonance imaging of the abnormal female pelvis. *AJR* 143:1259, 1984.
6. Gilbert, H. A., and Kagan, A. R. Metastases: Incidence, Detection, and Evaluation Without Histological Confirmation. In L. Weiss (Ed.). *Fundamental Aspects of Metastasis.* Amsterdam: North Holland Publishing Company, 1976. Chap. 23.
7. Goldhirsch, A., Triller, J. K., Greiner, R., et al. Computed tomography prior to second-look operation in advanced ovarian cancer. *Obstet. Gynecol.* 62:630, 1983.
8. Gordon, R. E., Mettler, F. A., Jr., Wicks, J. D., et al. Chest x-rays and full lung tomograms in gynecologic malignancy. *Cancer* 52:559, 1983.
9. Greene, M. H., Clark, J. W., and Blayney, D. W. The epidemiology of ovarian cancer. *Semin. Oncol.* 11:209, 1984.
10. Mamtora, H., and Isherwood, I. Computed tomography in ovarian carcinoma: Patterns of disease and limitations. *Clin. Radiol.* 33:165, 1982.
11. Richardson, G. S., Scully, R. E., Najamosama, N., et al. Common epithelial cancer of the ovary. *N. Engl. J. Med.* 312:415, 1985.
12. Whitley, N., Brenner, D., Francis, A., et al. Use of the computed tomographic whole body scanner to stage and follow patients with advanced ovarian carcinoma. *Invest. Radiol.* 16:479, 1981.

Cervical Carcinoma: Initial Staging

William D. Kaplan and Ross S. Berkowitz

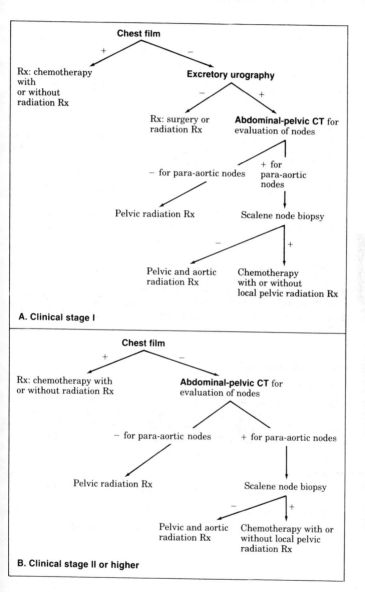

Chest film

+ → Rx: chemotherapy with or without radiation Rx

− → **Excretory urography**

   − → Rx: surgery or radiation Rx

   + → **Abdominal-pelvic CT** for evaluation of nodes

     − for para-aortic nodes → Pelvic radiation Rx

     + for para-aortic nodes → Scalene node biopsy

       − → Pelvic and aortic radiation Rx

       + → Chemotherapy with or without local pelvic radiation Rx

A. Clinical stage I

Chest film

+ → Rx: chemotherapy with or without radiation Rx

− → **Abdominal-pelvic CT** for evaluation of nodes

   − for para-aortic nodes → Pelvic radiation Rx

   + for para-aortic nodes → Scalene node biopsy

     − → Pelvic and aortic radiation Rx

     + → Chemotherapy with or without local pelvic radiation Rx

B. Clinical stage II or higher

Individual having an abnormal Pap smear or cervical biopsy diagnostic of cervical cancer

Comments

Initial spread to the lungs occurs infrequently—essentially 0% in stage I, less than 1% in stage II, and about 5% in stages III and IV; chest radiographs are essential for baseline purposes, however [9]

Delineation of localized disease is important: Patients treated with local surgery or radiation therapy have high chance of cure. Radiation therapy requires CT for planning of portals.

Initial spread is usually to pelvic and para-aortic nodes, with frequency varying with stage of tumor; with stage IIIB disease, up to 35% have tumor in common iliac and periaortic nodes [2, 12]. Half the patients with pelvic nodes have para-aortic nodes.

Para-aortic nodal involvement is rare in the absence of pelvic nodal involvement

About 28% of patients with para-aortic nodal involvement will have scalene node involvement [4]; these patients need systemic in addition to localized (radiation therapy) treatment

Treatment failure is frequently associated with the presence of local bulky tumor mass as well as tumor in regional lymph nodes [2]; distal metastases also occur [12]

During follow-up new tumor-related findings were seen on chest radiographs in 6% of patients with normal films initially [13]

Follow-up chest radiographs and/or CT are performed yearly for 3 years

Excretory Urography

Comments

Useful as a prognostic indicator: Ureteral obstruction indicates worse prognosis [9] and, by definition, stage III disease

About 35% of patients with stage III disease show ureteral obstruction on excretory urogram [1, 7, 15]; only 2% of patients with "presumed" stage I disease have this finding

Sensitivity

No specific data: however, for obstruction, in general, high

Specificity

For showing normal ureteral system: more than *90%*

Computed Tomography (CT) of Abdomen and Pelvis

Comments

Detects nodal disease
Directly visualizes tumor
Helps plan radiation therapy portals

Sensitivity

For detecting disease in para-aortic lymph nodes: about *70%* [5]
in nodes larger than 0.5 cm
For detecting disease in pelvic lymph nodes: approaching *100%*
[5]
False negatives can occur
In the presence of microscopic disease

Comment

For palpable pelvic tumor, CT findings correlate poorly with
clinical findings

Specificity

In showing normal para-aortic area: greater than *90%* [5]
In showing normal pelvic area: lower, between *50* and *75%* [5,
16]
False positives can occur
Because of hyperplastic nodes without tumor

Contribution of Magnetic Resonance Imaging [3, 6]

Provides an excellent demonstration of pelvic anatomy, para-
metrial extension, and if present, metastatic lymphadenopathy

References

1. Abayomi, O., Dritschilo, A., Emami, B., et al. The value of "routine tests" in the staging evaluation of gynecologic malignancies: A cost effectiveness analysis. *Int. J. Radiat. Oncol. Biol. Phys.* 8:241, 1982.
2. Berman, M. L., Keys, H., Creasman, W., et al. Survival and patterns of recurrence in cervical cancer metastatic to periaortic lymph nodes. *Gynecol. Oncol.* 19:8, 1984.
3. Bies, J. R., Ellis, J. H., Kopecky, K. K., et al. Assessment of primary gynecologic malignancies: Comparison of 0.15 T resistive MRI with CT. *AJR* 143:1249, 1984.
4. Brandt, B., III, and Lifshitz, S. Scalene node biopsy in advanced carcinoma of the cervix uteri. *Cancer* 47:1920, 1981.
5. Brenner, D. E., Whitley, N. O., Prempree, T., et al. An evaluation of the computed tomographic scanner for the staging of carcinoma of the cervix. *Cancer* 50:2323, 1982.

6. Butler, H., Bryan, P. J., LiPuma, J. P., et al. Magnetic resonance imaging of the abnormal female pelvis. *AJR* 143:1259, 1984.

7. Deale, C. J. C., and Du Toit, J. P. Routine investigations in the clinical staging of invasive carcinoma of the cervix: A critical evaluation. *S. Afr. Med. J.* 58:895, 1980.

8. Fenoglio, C. M., and Ferenczy, A. Etiologic factors in cervical neoplasia. *Semin. Oncol.* 9:349, 1982.

9. Gal, D., and Buchsbaum, H. J. The Staging of Cervical Carcinoma. In J. J. Sciarra (Ed.). *Gynecology and Obstetrics*. Philadelphia: Harper and Row, 1982. Vol. 4, Chap. 7, Pp. 1–7.

10. Gusberg, S. B., and Deppe, G. The earliest diagnosis of cervical cancer and its precursors. *Semin. Oncol.* 9:280, 1982.

11. Lagasse, L. D., Ballon, S. C., Berman, M. L., et al. Pretreatment lymphangiography and operative evaluation in carcinoma of the cervix. Am. J. Obstet. Gynecol. 134:219, 1979.

12. Nelson, J. H., Jr., Boyce, J., Macasaet, M., et al. Incidence, significance, and follow-up of para-aortic lymph node metastases in late invasive carcinoma of the cervix. *Am. J. Obstet. Gynecol.* 128:336, 1977.

13. Parker, R. G., and Friedman, R. F. A critical evaluation of the roentgenologic examination of patients with carcinoma of the cervix. *AJR* 96:100, 1966.

14. Photopulos, G. J., Shirley, R. E. L., Jr., and Ansbacher, R. Evaluation of conventional diagnostic tests for detection of recurrent carcinoma of the cervix. *Am. J. Obstet. Gynecol.* 129:533, 1977.

15. van Nagell, J. R., Jr., Sprague, A. D., and Roddick, J. W., Jr. The effect of intravenous pyelography and cystoscopy on the staging of cervical cancer. *Gynecol. Oncol.* 3:87, 1975.

16. Walsh, J. W., Amendola, M. A., Konerding, K. F., et al. Computed tomographic detection of pelvic and inguinal lymph-node metastases from primary and recurrent pelvic malignant disease. *Radiology* 137:157, 1980.

Uterine Sarcoma: Initial Staging

William D. Kaplan and Ross S. Berkowitz

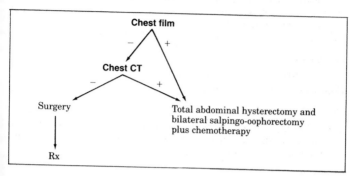

Typical Patient/Disorder

Individual with a sarcoma arising from any of the connective tissue elements of uterine structures or from the myometrium, endometrium, and blood vessels

Comments

At presentation, about 50% of patients have tumor confined to the corpus of the uterus (stage I) [7]

During follow-up period, about 50% of patients fail because of distant metastases only, and 50% fail because of distant and pelvic disease [7]

During follow-up, chest radiographs and CT of the abdomen are performed every 3 months for a year

Plain Chest Film

Studies comparing chest radiographs to CT in various tumors have found, on average, that 35% of patients with normal chest films will have abnormal CT [5]

Sensitivity

For detecting metastatic lung nodules: low; chest radiographs detect fewer nodules than CT by a factor of 0.3 [8]; resolution for nodules is about 4 mm

Specificity

For showing normal lungs: very high. Because of a low false positive ratio, metastatic disease is usually found in more than 90% of resected nodules seen on chest radiographs

Chest Computed Tomography (CT)

Excellent for visualizing the mediastinum (but in this tumor parenchyma is more heavily involved)
Better than chest films for detecting nodules, particularly pleural or subpleural
Provides very good resolution of nodules (4 mm)

Drawbacks

Cannot differentiate benign from malignant nodules
Potential contrast reaction

Sensitivity

For detecting metastatic nodules: high; CT detects more than 3 times as many nodules as does routine chest radiography and nearly 2 times as many as conventional tomography

Specificity

For showing normal lung parenchyma: moderate and lower than that of chest radiographs and conventional whole lung tomography. Its false positive ratio is such that among nodules seen on CT and resected at surgery, only 66% have metastases.

Abdominal Computed Tomography (CT)

Used for follow-up
Of the distant failure, most involve lung (60%) or upper abdomen (omentum, bowel, liver, etc.—70%); bone and brain occur rarely [6]

Drawbacks

Cannot identify microscopic disease

Sensitivity

No specific data are available for follow-up, but the information below offers some perspective:
    Compared to findings at surgery: CT agreed 84% of the time (16 of 19 patients); the remaining 16% were understaged [9]
False negatives can occur in
    Microscopic nodal disease
    Microscopic bladder involvement

Specificity

No specific data are available for follow-up, but the information below offers some perspective:
    Very high: No patients (0 out of 10) with tumors confined to corpus or cervix at surgery had CT suggesting extension [9]

Contribution of Magnetic Resonance Imaging [1, 3]

Defines wall invasion and extension to adjacent pelvic organs
Probably better at differentiation than CT or ultrasound

References

1. Bies, J. R., Ellis, J. H., Kopecky, K. K., et al. Assessment of primary gynecologic malignancies: Comparison of 0.15 T resistive MRI with CT. *AJR* 143:1249, 1984.
2. Enterline, H. T. Histopathology of sarcomas. *Semin. Oncol.* 8:133, 1981.
3. Hricak, H., Alpers, C., Crooks, L. E., et al. Magnetic resonance imaging of the female pelvis: Initial experience. *AJR* 141:1119, 1983.
4. Mintzer, R. A., Malave, S. R., Neiman, H. L. et al. Computed vs. conventional tomography in evaluation of primary and secondary pulmonary neoplasms. *Radiology* 132:653, 1979.
5. Muhm, J. R., Brown, L. R., and Crowe, J. K. Use of computed tomography in the detection of pulmonary nodules. *Mayo Clin. Proc.* 52:345, 1977.
6. Salazar, O. M., Bonfiglio, T. A., Patten, S. F., et al. Uterine sarcomas—analysis of failures with special emphasis on the use of adjuvant radiation therapy. *Cancer* 42:1161, 1978.
7. Salazar, O. M., Bonfiglio, T. A., Patten, S. F., et al. Uterine sarcomas—natural history, treatment and prognosis. *Cancer* 42:1152, 1978.
8. Schaner, E. G., Chang, A. E., Doppman, J. L., et al. Comparison of computed and conventional whole lung tomography in detecting pulmonary nodules: A prospective radiologic-pathologic study. *AJR* 131:51, 1978,.
9. Walsh, J. W., and Goplerud, D. R. Computed tomography of primary, persistent, and recurrent endometrial malignancy. *AJR* 139:1149, 1982.

Gestational Trophoblastic Tumor (GTT): Initial Staging

William D. Kaplan and Ross S. Berkowitz

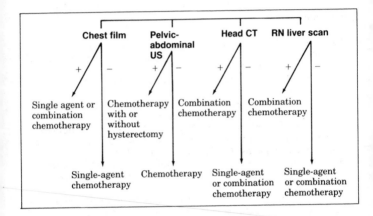

Typical Patient/Disorder

Young woman, recently pregnant, with bleeding or pelvic mass, discovered to represent malignant tumor of uterus

Comments

Gestational trophoblastic tumor applies to several tumor types—hydatidiform mole, invasive mole, and choriocarcinoma

Patients with locally invasive disease or distant disease confined to lungs are usually curable

Patients with disease in several sites (brain, liver) need multimodal therapy in order to have chance at cure; hence, the importance of accurate initial staging in this disease

The most common metastatic sites are lungs (80%), vagina or pelvis (20–30%), liver (10%), and brain (10%) [5].

After initial treatment, follow-up evaluation centers on human chorionic gonadotropin (HCG) levels. All patients are tested weekly until samples are normal for 3 consecutive weeks; tests are then performed monthly until normal for at least 12 consecutive months. Pelvic arteriography is required occasionally as well.

Plain Chest Film

Demonstrates pulmonary nodules (occurring in 45–87% of patients with metastatic disease) [2, 9], the differences being probably a function of the disease state

Nodules are metastatic until proven otherwise
Most lesions are parenchymal (70–92%); pleural or mediastinal involvement rare (less than 10%) [2, 9]

Sensitivity

For detecting metastatic lung nodules: low; chest radiographs
detect fewer nodules than either CT or whole lung tomography by factors of 0.3 and 0.5, respectively; resolution for nodules is about 4 mm

Specificity

For showing normal lungs: very high; because of low false positive ratio metastatic disease is usually found in more than
90% of resected nodules seen on chest radiography

Pelvic-Abdominal Ultrasound (US)

Evaluates primary tumor site as well as adjacent areas; can detect associated adnexal ovarian theca-lutein cysts
Provides secondary information about liver metastases, hydronephrosis, and hydroureter
May detect extensive uterine tumor involvement and help select
patients who may benefit from hysterectomy

Comments

Requires a full bladder

Sensitivity

For identifying persistent trophoblastic tumor: *74%* [4]
False negatives can occur
    In the presence of microscopic disease

Specificity

For showing normal uterus: approaching *100%* [4]

Head Computed Tomography (CT)

See Chapter 30, page 154, for detailed description

Comments

The incidence of central nervous system metastases from GTT
varies from 4–10% [12]; about half present prior to treatment
[1]
Brain metastases seldom occur prior to lung metastases [1]

Sensitivity

For detecting intracranial masses, tumors in particular: *95–
98%* [3]

False negatives can occur with
    Small lesions to the bony calvarium

Specificity

For showing normal intracranial structures or benign disease in patients suspected of malignant tumor, using contrast enhanced scans: *97%* [3]

For showing normal intracranial structures or benign disease in patients suspected of malignant tumor, using noncontrast enhanced scans: *97%* [3]

Radionuclide (RN) Liver-Spleen Scan

See Chapter 47, page 240, for detailed description

Comments

Liver metastases rarely occur before lung metastases

Up to 10% of patients may present with liver metastases [7]

Metastatic disease to the liver usually presents as focal rather than diffuse disease; hence all imaging modalities (e.g., radionuclide liver scans, ultrasound, CT) are relatively sensitive

Sensitivity

For detecting GTT lesions metastatic to the liver: about *87%*, perhaps higher

Specificity

No specific data: probably about *80%*

False positives can occur
    If heterogeneous patterns are considered abnormal
    More than 80% of newly diagnosed patients have liver scans showing heterogeneous uptake; this is presumably secondary to hormonal or chemotherapeutic effects [12]

Pelvic Angiography

Identifies sites of resistant uterine tumor to aid in deciding between surgical approaches of total abdominal hysterectomy or subsegmental resection

Drawbacks

Vascular abnormalities persist even after remission: thus, method may not be as good for following response to therapy [6, 8]

Potential allergic reaction to contrast, with complications (e.g., nausea, vomiting) possible

Sensitivity

No published data; however, for defining intrauterine tumor our data suggest high

Specificity

No exact data, but likely high
False positives can occur
> If there is an increase in uterine vascularization from other causes (e.g., normal pregnancy, missed abortion, retained benign molar tissue) [8]

Contribution of Magnetic Resonance Imaging [13]

Demonstrates the gross morphological features of neoplasms
Useful in detecting invasive trophoblastic disease

References

1. Athanassiou, A., Begent, R. H. J., Newlands, E. S., et al. Central nervous system metastases of choriocarcinoma: 23 years' experience at Charing Cross Hospital. *Cancer* 52:1728, 1983.
2. Bagshawe, K. D., and Garnett, E. S. Radiological changes in the lungs of patients with trophoblastic tumors. *Br. J. Radiol.* 36:673, 1963.
3. Baker, H. L., Jr., Houser, O. W., and Campbell, J. K. National Cancer Institute study: Evaluation of computed tomography in the diagnosis of intracranial neoplasms. I. Overall results. *Radiology* 136:91, 1980.
4. Berkowitz, R. S., Birnholz, J., Goldstein, D. P., et al. Pelvic ultrasonography and the management of gestational trophoblastic disease. *Gynecol. Oncol.* 15:403, 1983.
5. Berkowitz, R. S., and Goldstein, D. P. Gestational Trophoblastic Tumors. In B. Eiseman, W. A. Robinson, and G. Steele (Eds.). *Follow-up of the Cancer Patient.* New York: Thieme-Stratton, 1982. Chap. 31.
6. Brewis, R. A. L., and Bagshawe, K. D. Pelvic arteriography in invasive trophoblastic neoplasia. *Br. J. Radiol.* 41:481, 1968.
7. Goldstein, D. P., and Berkowitz, R. S. *Gestational Trophoblastic Neoplasms: Clinical Principles of Diagnosis and Management.* Philadelphia: Saunders, 1982.
8. Levin, D. C., Staiano, S., Schneider, M., et al. Complementary role of sonography and arteriography in management of uterine choriocarcinoma. *AJR* 125:462, 1975.
9. Libshitz, H. I., Baber, C. E., and Hammond, C. B. The pulmonary metastases of choriocarcinoma. *Obstet. Gynecol.* 49:412, 1977.
10. Mandybur, T. I. Intracranial hemorrhage caused by metastatic tumors. *Neurology* 27:650, 1977.
11. Smith, T. J., Kemeny, M. M., Sugarbaker, P. H., et al. A prospective study of hepatic imaging in the detection of metastatic disease. *Ann. Surg.* 195:486, 1982.
12. Sumers, E. H., Berkowitz, R. S., Wang, A.-M., et al. Radiocolloid scintigraphy and cranial computed tomography in staging gestational trophoblastic disease. *Radiology.* In press, 1985.
13. Weinreb, J. C., Lowe, T. W., Santos-Ramos, R., et al. Magnetic resonance imaging in obstetric diagnosis. *Radiology* 154:157, 1985.

Appendixes

Definitions

Abdomen, upright film Film exposed while patient stands upright with diaphragm included in the examination so as to detect free air as well as air-fluid levels in the intestine.

Abdominal CT See *CT*

Abscess drainage, percutaneous Needle inserted into the region of interest and replaced by a catheter with drainage of abscess.

Air contrast examination Commonly used in the examination of the colon. Involves instillation first of some barium and then of air so that the barium coats the mucosa of the intestine while the gas distends the bowel loops. Polyps and carcinoma of the colon will have a coating of barium and are seen in fine detail against the surrounding gas-filled lumen.

Angiography The study of the vascular bed using contrast agents. Includes both arteriography and venography. A highly concentrated solution of an organic iodinated molecule is injected rapidly in adequate volume to opacify a particular vascular bed. Image is generally recorded either on a rapid cut-film changer or on motion picture studies.

> *Aortography* Thoracic, lumbar, or thoracolumbar aortic visualization, usually by transfemoral catheter passage to the region of interest, rapid contrast injection.
>
> *Selective Arteriography* Precurved catheter placed in the vessel that supplies the vascular bed in question. For example, with GI bleeding, selective mesenteric and celiac arteriography is usually performed to identify the bleeding site.
>
> *Peripheral Venography* Injection of a large volume of contrast agent into foot veins with fluoroscopic monitoring and careful follow-up of venous filling; spot films and/or overhead films record presence of thrombus, occlusion, varices.
>
> *Renal Venography* Curved catheter is inserted through femoral vein and inferior vena cava into the renal vein. Contrast agent is injected retrograde against the stream so as to opacify the main renal vein and its branches. Best accomplished if a small volume of norepinephrine is injected first into the renal artery so as to slow flow during venography.
>
> *Inferior Venacavography* Catheters inserted in both common iliac veins and 40 to 45 ml of contrast agent injected rapidly under pressure with film recording.

AP and lateral radiographs See *X-rays, conventional*

Arterial DSA See *DSA*

Arteriography See *Angiography*

Arthrography Visualization of a joint by injection of gas and/or contrast medium and radiographic exposures in multiple projections.

Barium enema See *BE*

Barium esophagraphy A procedure in which the patient swallows a barium sulfate mixture, the course of which is observed fluoroscopically by the radiologist, with recording of the image on films.

Barium swallow See *Barium esophagraphy*

BE (Barium Enema) Barium instilled into the colon with the patient in the supine position and its course followed under fluoroscopy. Frequent changes in position so as to maximize information about the flexures of the colon. Barium fills the colon at high pressure, and the examination is not complete until the cecum is filled. Optimally reflux through the ileocecal valve into the terminal ileum. Spot films taken during fluoroscopy and overhead conventional films are obtained.

Bone scan Tc-99m methylene diphosphonate (MDP) injected intravenously and imaging of skeletal system begun 3 hours later. Total body imaging requires 45–60 minutes; companion radiographs of abnormal areas required.

Brain scan Tc-99m, in the form of pertechnetate or glucoheptonate, injected intravenously and images begun 1–2 hours later. Forty-five minutes required with pretreatment with perchlorate if pertechnetate used. In some patients flow study is done initially—images taken every second or so during the first transit through the cerebral circulation.

Cardiac catheterization Catheter is inserted into the venous and arterial system and under fluoroscopic control is passed into the chambers of the heart and pulmonary artery, with concurrent pressure measurements and frequently angiocardiography as well.

Cardiac ultrasound See *Ultrasound*

Cerebral angiography See *Angiography*

Cervical spine x-rays See *X-rays, conventional*

Chest fluoroscopy See *Fluoroscopy*

Chest CT See *CT*

Chest x-rays See *X-rays, conventional*

Cholecystography, oral Contrast agent (usually Telepaque) given orally about 14 hours before the examination. With its absorption and excretion through the liver, it ultimately fills and opacifies the gallbladder, the cystic duct, and the common bile duct in normal subjects. Now used infrequently because ultrasound and hepatobiliary studies have proved to be so useful.

Cholescintigraphy or hepatobiliary study DISIDA labeled with Tc-99m injected intravenously in fasting patient (at least 3–4 hours) and sequential imaging begun immediately to evaluate transit through liver into gallbladder and GI tract. Images taken for 90 minutes with delayed (at 4 hours) images necessary to help distinguish acute from chronic cholecystitis.

Colonoscopy Endoscopy of the colon, usually done with fiberoptic flexible colonoscope.

CT (computed tomography, "CAT scanning") A radiographic method in which a fine beam of x-rays traverses an anatomical area with the remnant radiation (that which is not absorbed or attenuated) recorded and subsequently digitized. By use of multiple projections and a series of complex equations, the computer organizes the information reflecting the attentuation of various tissues into a coherent cross-sectional image.

Computed tomography of bone See *CT*

Computed tomography of the liver See *CT*

Computed tomography of thorax See *CT*

Conventional tomography See *Tomography*

CT of abdomen and pelvis See *CT*

CT of chest and abdomen See *CT*

CT of pelvis and retroperitoneum See *CT*

Cyst puncture Fine needle is inserted under fluoroscopic, ultrasound, or CT guidance, and a sample of fluid is obtained from the cyst. Cyst opacification by contrast injection at times. Previously most commonly performed in renal cysts, but now used less frequently for that purpose because of information from CT. May be done in any cystic structure.

Cystography Filling of the bladder with contrast agent inserted through urethral catheterization, with fluoroscopic and radiographic examination to detect abnormalities of the bladder.

DSA (digital subtraction angiography) A method of recording the appearance of contrast agent in the cardiovascular system in which the image amplified fluoroscopic system is digitized, processed, and recreated with heightened visibility of the vascular bed being examined.

Dual photon absorptiometry See *Photon absorptiometry*

Echocardiogram See *Ultrasound*

Endoscopic retrograde cholangiopancreatography See *ERCP*

Endoscopy Employs a tube with highly developed optics to enable direct vision of important areas of the gastrointestinal tract, trachea, bronchus, and other hollow organs. Usually performed by the gastroenterologist or surgeon rather than by the radiologist.

Enteroclysis A special technique for studying the small bowel; a catheter is passed through the oral cavity, esophagus, and stomach into the small intestine as a means of injecting adequate volumes of barium rapidly (over a period of 15 minutes or so) so as to distend and depict the small intestine clearly. Because contrast agent is delivered in the small intestine, coating is usually excellent.

ERCP (endoscopic retrograde cholangiopancreatography) A method whereby intubation of the common duct or the pancreatic duct is attained via passage of the tube through the esophagus, stomach, and duodenum into the ampulla of Vater. Once in place, contrast is injected and opacifies more or less of the common duct and pancreatic duct as well as some of the branches.

Excretory urography Sequential examination of the kidneys, ureter, and bladder in which approximately 1 ml per kilo of a hyperosmotic iodinated organic molecule is injected intravenously, with planned filming thereafter. Initial films obtained early, and delayed when needed. Contrast opacifies renal parenchyma, collecting system of the kidney, ureters, and bladder.

Exretory urogram   See *Urography*

Fluoroscopy   The patient is examined in real-time using a fluoroscopic screen with image intensifier. A beam of x-rays passes through the patient, with the relative absorption reflected in the image visible on the output screen. Commonly used in the examination of the heart, gastrointestinal tract, and vascular system.

Gallium studies for infection   Gallium citrate is injected directly intravenously and images usually begun 48 hours later. Colon preparation used by many since gallium is excreted into the colon. Delayed views at 72 hours frequently necessary.

Gallium studies for staging or monitoring cancer patients   Same procedure as above except higher dose of gallium used; also, imaging usually delayed until 72 hours to minimize soft-tissue activity.

GI bleeding study   Tc-99m labeled to patient's own red blood cells used; imaging begun immediately over abdomen and continued for 90 minutes. Patients with negative studies examined again at 24 hours.

Head CT   See *CT*

Hepatic ultrasound   See *Ultrasound*

Indium WBC study for infection   Patient's white cells obtained (about 50–100 ml whole blood taken) and labeled in vitro with indium oxine. Imaging of suspected areas begun at 24 hours, occasionally earlier.

Intravenous digital subtraction angiography (IV DSA)   See *DSA*

Joint aspiration   Needle is inserted into a joint, frequently under fluoroscopic guidance, with removal of fluid for culture, cell count, and smear. In most instances this is followed by arthrography.

KUB   See *Plain film of abdomen*

Lower limb phlebography   See *Angiography, Venography*

Lumbar spine CT   See *CT*

Lung scan: perfusion   Particles (25 micron) of macroaggregated albumin labeled with Tc-99m injected intravenously. Particles block about 0.1% of precapillary arterioles and measure regional pulmonary perfusion.

Lung scan: ventilation   Several techniques and materials possible. Commonly done with xenon-133 which patient inhales, then rebreathes for 2 minutes in closed system, and then washes out. Areas of match or mismatch evaluated on initial inhalation and areas of trapping as evidence of chronic lung disease evaluated on delayed images.

Lymphangiography   The study of the lymph vessels and lymph nodes using iodinated oils as a contrast agent, injected into the peripheral lymphatics of the foot. The transit of the oil is followed, with x-rays of the channels obtained shortly after injection, and node architecture visualized 24 hours later.

Mammography   Radiographic method of obtaining x-ray images of the breast at acceptable dose levels both for disease detection initially and later as a baseline for comparison during follow-up. Ultrasound, CT, and nuclear magnetic resonance mammography may be used for specific supplementary information but are not of proven superiority to x-ray mammography.

Meckel's study (for diverticulum)   Tc-99m pertechnetate injected intravenously and images begun immediately over abdomen. Meckel's diverticulum, like normal gastric mucosa, concentrates pertechnetate. Imaging takes 1 hour.

Metrizamide myelography   See *Myelography*

Myelography   Needle inserted into the subarachnoid space through the posterior intervertebral space, with the injection of contrast agent, usually metrizamide. The patient is manipulated so that the contrast agent flows to different levels while films are obtained that demonstrate contours of spinal cord and nerve roots. The method accurately depicts the subarachnoid space, defines extra dural and intradural (intramedullary or extramedullary) abnormalities, and localizes the level of compression, if present.

Oblique films   See *X-rays, conventional*

Oral cholecystography   See *Cholecystography, oral*

PA and lateral chest film   See *X-rays, conventional*

Pelvic and abdominal ultrasound   See *Ultrasound*

Pelvic angiography   See *Angiography*

Percutaneous transhepatic cholangiography   See *PTC*

Photon absorptiometry   For single photon absorptiometry long bone, usually distal radius, placed in front of radioactive source (usually iodine-125). For dual photon absorptiometry, vertebra or entire skeleton placed in front of radioactive source (usually gadolinium-153). Bone mineral content measured via transmission of emitted photons.

Plain films   See *X-rays, conventional*

Plain film of abdomen   Conventional anterior/posterior view of the abdomen; frequently accompanied by a lateral film, obtained at 90° to the anterior/posterior. A complete examination may also include an upright film, in order to detect fluid levels or air beneath the diaphragm or decubitus films.

PTC (percutaneous transhepatic cholangiography)   Percutaneous needle entry into the liver through which a wire is passed; the needle is removed and the catheter is threaded over the wire into the biliary tree. Contrast agent is injected through the catheter. Defines the presence and location of obstruction or abnormalities in the biliary and/or pancreatic ducts.

Pulmonary angiography   See *Angiography*

Radionuclide liver scan   Colloidal particles labeled with Tc-99m injected intravenously and imaging begun 15 minutes later. Allows assessment of reticuloendothelial function.

Radionuclide renal study   Done with one of several possible agents, all using Tc-99m. DMSA serves as best agent for assessing cortical mass and morphology; DTPA for evaluating collecting systems; glucoheptonate for evaluating renal parenchyma and collecting systems; DMSA for visualizing columns of Bertin.

Radionuclide scrotal scan   Tc-99m pertechnetate injected intravenously and flow study obtained for 60 seconds or so. Several static images taken with pinhole collimator.

RBC study for hemangiomas in liver   Tc-99m labeled to patient's own red blood cells used; imaging begun immediately with dynamic flow study. Static views taken at 10 minutes and then at 30–40 minutes. Hemangiomas show increased activity on late images but not on early ones.

Renal angiography   See *Angiography*

Renal scintigraphy using Tc-99m DMSA or Tc-99m glucoheptonate   See *Radionuclide renal study*

Renal vein sampling   Selective renal vein catheterization from the femoral vein with collection of blood samples for renin assay.

Retrograde pyelogram   Done during cystoscopy. Contrast injected into ureteral orifices and films of abdomen taken.

Small bowel examination   Barium given by mouth fills the small intestine. Fluoroscopy and serial films at intervals record the appearance of small bowel loops.

Spine CT   See *CT*

Thallium study   For a combined exercise and rest study, patient is exercised on treadmill and thallous chloride (a potassium analog) injected at end of exercise level achieved. Images taken immediately and then again at 4 hours. Latter images help distinguish infarction from ischemia.

Thoracic aortography   See *Aortography*

Thoracic CT   See *CT*

Thyroid scan   Tc-99m pertechnetate injected intravenously; acts as iodide analog. Imaging begun after 20 minutes and takes 40 minutes; proper study requires that palpable nodules be correlated with scan.

Tomography   Sectional radiographs in which the volumes above and below the level of the plane of interest are deliberately blurred, while the plane of interest, because it fails to exhibit significant motion, may be seen with great precision.

UGI (upper gastrointestinal series)   Barium swallowed by mouth so as to visualize the esophagus, the stomach, the duodenum, and the small intestine. An interactive examination with the fluoroscopist responsible for recording abnormalities on spot films. Conventional overhead films are also obtained.

Urethrography   Radiographic examination of the urethra with a contrast agent. Contrast may be injected in retrograde fashion or excreted from contrast-filled bladder.

US (Ultrasound)   A transducer projects an ultrasound beam into a given area or a particular viscus. The echoes are captured and depicted in a reflection of both normal and abnormal viscera. Useful in the examination of the abdomen, in pregnancy, and in cardiac evaluation.

Vertebral CT   See *CT*

X-rays, conventional examinations

AP (Anteroposterior) A view in which the beam is at right angles to the coronal plane and the anterior portion of the patient is closest to the x-ray beam.

Lateral A view at 90° to the anteroposterior.

Obliques Films exposed to right or left of the anteroposterior plane. May reveal abnormalities not readily apparent on AP or lateral film.

B

Magnetic Resonance Imaging

Ferenc A. Jolesz

Magnetic resonance imaging (MRI) is a new diagnostic imaging modality emerging from the stage of basic science applications and rapidly developing into a method comparable to existing techniques, such as ultrasound and computed tomography (CT). Its potential for widespread clinical use seems clear; the unique information MR signals provide may represent an important step in the diagnostic evaluation of a number of disease processes. Not only is detailed anatomical information obtained with good spatial resolution, but chemical and physiological data may be provided as well.

MRI is a complex method. Its imaging principles are more interrelated with the physical behavior of the imaged object than is the case with x-ray imaging. MRI does not measure attenuation—as do x-ray methods—but rather nuclear motion in a magnetic field, with time the important parameter. Proton MRI measures proton density and T1–T2 relaxation times, which in tissues are closely related not only to water and lipid content but to water compartmentalization, membrane surface, diffusion, and several other parameters. Such properties of normal and pathological tissues are not well defined. Furthermore, we do not fully understand how the structural organization of water in cells influences the MR parameters or how other nonwater molecules, mainly macromolecules, influence the structure and thus the mobility of water.

Nonetheless, MRI has a remarkable ability to delineate cross-sectional and three-dimensional anatomy in multiple planes. Multiplanar imaging is especially well adapted to visualizing cardiac anatomy, the mediastinum, and the brain. An impressive feature of MRI is its capacity to depict the cardiac chambers and the major blood vessels without using contrast media. It may be particularly useful in demonstrating vascular anatomy and blood flow simultaneously. Despite early enthusiasm, spectroscopic studies indicate that MRI has failed as yet to demonstrate specificity in differentiating malignant from benign tissue. On the other hand, it appears to be highly sensitive in distinguishing normal from pathological tissues; edema, necrosis, and benign and malignant neoplasms may demonstrate similar characteristics.

MRI has earned its highest level of clinical credibility in the central nervous system (CNS). Cerebral and spinal MRI has considerable diagnostic potential, and several advantages are already apparent. Its multiplanar images and absence of artifacts permit excellent anatomical delineation of different intracranial and intraspinal lesions, including some poorly demonstrated by CT. Of particular interest are the lesions found in multiple sclerosis and other demyelinating diseases. The sensitivity of MRI in detecting white matter lesions, even in previously "hidden" areas such as the brain stem or the spinal cord, may prove to be of great value.

Imaging or detecting nuclei other than protons represents a potentially rewarding direction for research. Metabolic changes in active organs like muscle can be followed by phosphorus MR spectroscopy. Relative measurement of ATP and creatine phosphate levels or intracellular pH provides valuable information about the effect of exercise on muscle. Metabolic defects can also be detected. Sodium imaging or spectroscopy may show changes in tissue permeability and viability. Thus, the degree of damage or improvement may be tracked noninvasively in several pathophysiological processes, such as myocardial infarct and epilepsy.

The state of the art is rapidly changing in clinical MRI; instrumentation development continues and obsolescence must be anticipated. Despite some obvious limitations, it is clear that MRI will represent an important part of diagnostic imaging. Finding optimal imaging strategies is the principal task of the radiologist, and the effectiveness of diagnostic MRI will depend on those strategies. MRI's ultimate roles are yet to be discovered, and MRI research has become a fruitful area of medical activity.

Dose to Critical Organs

Philip F. Judy and Robert E. Zimmerman

This appendix is divided into two parts: doses from conventional radiographs and doses from nuclear medicine procedures. Doses for conventional films were estimated using the techniques in operation at the Brigham and Women's Hospital. Those for nuclear medicine procedures were calculated using the indicated injected doses. Doses from CT assume no contrast. If contrast is used, then all doses need to be increased in approximate proportion to the number and location of additional cuts. All doses are given in millirads rather than the conventional rads or fraction of rads. For the uninitiated reader, it must be emphasized that 1 rad equals 1000 mrad, and that the background dose that we all receive per annum (on average) is about 200 mrad, or 0.2 rad.

Doses from Conventional Radiographs

Angiography

	mrad
Abdominal angiography	
Maximum skin	37000
Testes	900
Ovaries	7000
Red bone marrow	2800
Thyroid	<1
Uterus	7000
Cerebral angiography	
Maximum skin	17000
Testes	<1
Ovaries	<1
Red bone marrow	500
Thyroid	4000
Uterus	<1
Coronary angiography	
Maximum skin	28000
Testes	20
Ovaries	30
Red bone marrow	1800
Thyroid	1800
Uterus	30
Superior mesenteric angiography	
Maximum skin	11000
Testes	10
Ovaries	100
Red bone marrow	2000
Thyroid	50
Uterus	100

Arthrography of hip

Maximum skin	500
Testes	80
Ovaries	120
Red bone marrow	40
Thyroid	<1
Uterus	300

Barium enema

Maximum skin	11000
Testes	300
Ovaries	2100
Red bone marrow	800
Thyroid	<1
Uterus	1800

Chest

Chest (PA and lateral)
Maximum skin	50
Testes	<1
Ovaries	<1
Red bone marrow	4
Thyroid	10
Uterus	<1

Conventional whole lung tomography
Maximum skin	3600
Testes	<1
Ovaries	17
Red bone marrow	400
Thyroid	760
Uterus	16

Computed tomography (noncontrast)

Abdomen
Maximum skin	2200
Testes	90
Ovaries	950
Red bone marrow	500
Thyroid	2
Uterus	1100

Abdomen and pelvis
Maximum skin	4400
Testes	1000
Ovaries	1400
Red bone marrow	750
Thyroid	3
Uterus	1600

Femur
Maximum skin	3500
Testes	1000
Ovaries	50

Red bone marrow	60
Thyroid	<1
Uterus	60
Head	
Maximum skin	4500
Testes	<1
Ovaries	<1
Red bone marrow	200
Thyroid	800
Uterus	<1
Kidney	
Maximum skin	3500
Testes	70
Ovaries	700
Red bone marrow	375
Thyroid	2
Uterus	500
Spine, lumbar	
Maximum skin	4500
Testes	200
Ovaries	700
Red bone marrow	375
Thyroid	2
Uterus	700
Spine, thoracic	
Maximum skin	2500
Testes	<1
Ovaries	200
Red bone marrow	500
Thyroid	200
Uterus	20

Cystography

Maximum skin	1500
Testes	700
Ovaries	300
Red bone marrow	30
Thyroid	<1
Uterus	500

Digital subtraction angiography (DSA)

Renal	
Maximum skin	23000
Testes	500
Ovaries	1000
Red bone marrow	800
Thyroid	50
Uterus	800

Endoscopic retrograde cholangiopancreatography (ERCP)

Maximum skin	400
Testes	<1

Ovaries	2
Red bone marrow	20
Thyroid	<1
Uterus	2

Excretory urography

Maximum skin	4000
Testes	100
Ovaries	800
Red bone marrow	300
Thyroid	<1
Uterus	300

Intravenous cholangiography

Maximum skin	800
Testes	1
Ovaries	35
Red bone marrow	30
Thyroid	2
Uterus	30

KUB and upright of abdomen

Maximum skin	800
Testes	20
Ovaries	150
Red bone marrow	60
Thyroid	<1
Uterus	140

Lumbar spine

AP and lateral

Maximum skin	400
Testes	5
Ovaries	200
Red bone marrow	50
Thyroid	<1
Uterus	200

Complete lumbar series

Maximum skin	850
Testes	12
Ovaries	470
Red bone marrow	110
Thyroid	<1
Uterus	470

Lymphangiography

Maximum skin	2400
Testes	60
Ovaries	450
Red bone marrow	250
Thyroid	350
Uterus	450

Myelography

Cervical

Maximum skin	400
Testes	<1
Ovaries	<1
Red bone marrow	15
Thyroid	80
Uterus	<1

Lumbar

Maximum skin	1000
Testes	20
Ovaries	900
Red bone marrow	160
Thyroid	<1
Uterus	900

Percutaneous transhepatic cholangiography

Maximum skin	800
Testes	20
Ovaries	150
Red bone marrow	60
Thyroid	<1
Uterus	100

Retrograde pyelography

Maximum skin	2000
Testes	50
Ovaries	400
Red bone marrow	150
Thyroid	<1
Uterus	150

Skull series

Full

Maximum skin	250
Testes	<1
Ovaries	<1
Red bone marrow	20
Thyroid	150
Uterus	<1

Limited

Maximum skin	200
Testes	<1
Ovaries	<1
Red bone marrow	15
Thyroid	100
Uterus	<1

Spine radiographs: full series

Maximum skin	800
Testes	10

Ovaries	450
Thyroid	200
Red bone marrow	100
Uterus	400

Upper gastrointestinal series

Maximum skin	7000
Testes	1
Ovaries	12
Red bone marrow	200
Thyroid	5
Uterus	10

Doses from Nuclear Medicine Procedures

Bone scan (18 mCi Tc-99m MDP injected)

Testes	270
Ovaries	270
Red bone marrow	630
Bladder	1440
Kidney	540
Skeleton	720

Brain scan (25 mCi Tc-99m glucoheptonate injected)

Testes	95
Ovaries	170
Red bone marrow	300
Kidneys	7500

DISIDA (diisopropyl iminodiacetic acid) or hepatobiliary study (2 mCi Tc-99m DISIDA injected)

Testes	5
Ovaries	100
Red bone marrow	40
Liver	180
Upper large intestine	1100

Flow study for any organ (10 mCi Tc-99m DTPA injected)

Testes	50
Ovaries	70
Red bone marrow	95
Bladder wall	3500
Kidneys	900

Gallium scan for infection (5 mCi gallium citrate injected)

Testes	1200
Ovaries	1400
Red bone marrow	2900
Lower large intestine	4500

(For tumor imaging 10 mCi are usually injected; above doses are then doubled.)

Liver scan (3 mCi Tc-99m sulfur colloid injected)

Testes	4
Ovaries	20
Red bone marrow	9
Liver	1020
Spleen	630

Lung perfusion study (2.5 mCi of Tc-99m MAA injected)

Testes	12
Ovaries	20
Red Marrow	38
Liver	45
Lungs	550

Meckel's scan (10 mCi Tc-99m pertechnetate injected)

Testes	120
Ovaries	220
Red bone marrow	190
Stomach wall	2500
Thyroid	3400
Upper large intestine	1200

RBC study for heart or GI bleeding study (in vivo label, 20 mCi Tc-99m pertechnetate injected)

Testes	106
Ovaries	420
Red bone marrow	340
Heart	1100
Kidney	400
Liver	460
Lung	460
Spleen	540
Thyroid	420

Renal scan (5 mCi Tc-99m DMSA injected)

Testes	70
Ovaries	115
Red bone marrow	175
Kidneys	3750

Renal scan (10 mCi Tc-99m glucoheptonate injected)

Testes	38
Ovaries	69
Red bone marrow	120
Kidneys	3000

Thallium scan (2 mCi thallous chloride injected)

Testes	600
Ovaries	600
Red bone marrow	500
Heart	400
Kidneys	800

Thyroid scan (5 mCi Tc-99m pertechnetate injected)

Testes	60
Ovaries	110
Red bone marrow	95
Stomach wall	1250
Thyroid	1700
Upper large intestine wall	600

Xenon ventilation scan (20 mCi Xe-133 gas inhaled)

Testes	20
Ovaries	20
Red bone marrow	30
Lung	380
Tracheal mucosa	2100
Uterus	30

Charge Data

Accurate cost data for health services are difficult to obtain. Charge data are more available and hence can provide the reader with an *approximate* idea of the relative costs of certain radiological services. We caution the reader, however, to recognize that charges are poor substitutes for costs for two reasons. First, charge data have sometimes been developed in the light of marketplace considerations rather than of actual costs. Second, before prospective payment (and hence for most of the data collected during this survey) efforts to maximize reimbursement included selective price shifting; charges for certain ancillaries may have been increased if these resources were used primarily by patients who were insured by nonregulated charge payors. Thus, large differences in charges can be expected from hospital to hospital.

The following table attempts to give the reader some idea of the magnitude of charges for a number of relatively common and/or expensive examinations discussed in this book. We have included a few other miscellaneous examinations of potential interest as well.

The data were derived from a survey of eight teaching hospitals in different areas of the country. Both technical and professional fees are included. These figures should not be construed as the *correct* or *appropriate* charge or as a reflection of real *cost*. Instead, they are meant to inform the reader as to the variability of charges leveled in a small and specialized group of hospitals throughout the country.

Examination	Median Charge ($)	Range ($)
Conventional		
Barium enema		
Single contrast	205	145–220
Double contrast	232	195–281
Bones		
Femur	83	53–123
Forearm	63	52–116
Knees, both	117	74–155
Chest PA and lateral	64	42–91

Examination	Median Charge ($)	Range ($)
Cervical spine		
Two films	87	65–137
Four films	92	73–137
Excretion urography	185	167–240
KUB	64	48–106
Lumbar spine	104	78–136
Metastatic bone series	177	123–257
Upper gastrointestinal series	197	104–225
Ultrasound of abdomen	203	162–301
Special Procedures		
Angiography		
Carotid, unilateral	1145	442–1645
Coronary	1285	839–2210
Computed tomography		
Head, contrast	390	298–620
Head, no contrast	345	189–548
Body, contrast	509	342–654
Body, no contrast	435	189–616
Endoscopic retrograde cholangiopancreatography (ERCP)	224	166–588
Percutaneous transhepatic cholangiography	500	380–713
Nuclear Medicine		
Bone scan	330	244–507
Bone marrow scan	294	288–684
Brain scan	269	219–380
Hepatobiliary study	332	241–387
Liver scan	286	220–395
Lung scan, perfusion	274	200–414
Thallium, rest alone	355	288–654
Thallium, rest and exercise	440	358–794

Index

Index